At 9, Adro Sarnelli, an unknown kid from Sydney's western suburbs, was 75 kilograms (165 pounds) and fighting his way through childhood feeling angry and isolated, struggling with schoolyard taunts, low self-esteem and abuse. At 18, he was close to 120 kilograms (264 pounds) and trying to find his place in the world, putting everyone but himself first and using the 'no time' excuse for not dealing with his escalating weight. Then at 26, having failed with numerous diets, and weighing in excess of 150 kilograms (330 pounds), he made a decision to try one last time to lose the weight, and become the person and father he always wanted to be – fit, thin, happy and involved. On a whim, he auditioned for **The Biggest Loser**. Not only did he go on to win the reality TV show, inspiring millions of Australians by losing over 50 kilograms (110 pounds) in four months, he also discovered that he'd had the power within himself all along to create a **new me**.

AN IMPORTANT NOTE

Please bear in mind that the activities and suggestions in this book are for general information purposes only and may not be suitable for your particular circumstances. Before undertaking any weight loss program, making a change in your diet, or starting a new exercise program always consult with a qualified medical practitioner to ensure the program is compatible with your particular health situation and needs. The publisher and author exclude any liability for injury or loss arising from undertaking activities in this book. The New Me Program is intended for healthy adults, aged 18 and over. This book is solely for inspirational, informational and educational purposes and although every effort has been made to ensure that the contents of this book are accurate, it must not be treated as a substitute for qualified medical advice. Neither the author nor the publisher can be held responsible for any loss or claim arising out of the use, or misuse, of the suggestions made or the failure to take medical advice. The before and after profiles are real-life examples of weight loss at The New Me Weight Loss Retreat program, but everyone's circumstances are different and individual results, even when using the same program, may vary. But it's not all about me; I hope this book is a chance to change your life too. So grab a pen, I want you to use my story and my book as the beginning of your own success story.

A NOTE ON KILOJOULES AND CALORIES

Both kilojoules and calories are measures of energy. Kilojoules are part of the metric system commonly used in Australia but not in some other countries such as the US. That said, in this book I have used calories because it's what I got used to during *The Biggest Loser* and prefer to use. One calorie/cal is equivalent to 4.2 kilojoules/kJ. If you like to work in kilojoules, to convert the calorie measurements used throughout this book into kilojoules, simply multiply the calorie measurement by 4.2. For example, to convert 100 calories to kilojoules: 100 x 4.2 = 420kJ.

THE
NEW ME

Eat Smart • Move More • Think Thin

ADRO SARNELLI

with Donna Jones

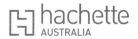

hachette
AUSTRALIA

Published in Australia and New Zealand in 2010
by Hachette Australia
(An imprint of Hachette Australia Pty Limited)
Level 17, 207 Kent Street, Sydney NSW 2000
www.hachette.com.au

National Library of Australia
Cataloguing-in-Publication data

Sarnelli, Adro

The new me / Adro Sarnelli.

9780733624216 (pbk.)

Sarnelli, Adro.
Weight loss.
Exercise.
Physical fitness.
Health.

613.25

Front cover design: Blue Cork Design
Front cover photographs: Michael Moynihan Photography
Internal design: Judi Rowe, Agave Creative Group
Internal photographs courtesy of Adro Sarnelli except where indicated otherwise
Printed in Australia by Griffin Press an Accredited ISO AS/NZS
14001:2004 Environmental Management System printer.

To my amazing children,
Odessa Jane and Eden Harper,
without you I would be nothing
and for you I will be everything.

For Eligh
Hopefully your eleven weeks here
were enough to make you want
to come back one day.
In our hearts forever.
26/6/07–15/9/07.

Contents

PART 3: The New Me Program *Planning and preparing for The New You*

PART 4: The New Me Tool Kit *Putting the program into practice to build The New You*

About the authors

Following his achievement on *The Biggest Loser*, **Adro Sarnelli** gained extensive national media coverage. He has been featured in *Who Weekly, Women's Weekly, Men's Health* and a variety of weight loss magazines, as well as television appearances on shows including *Today Tonight, A Current Affair, Rove Live* and *Today*. Adro's numerous radio interviews have aired on almost every major station in the country. *The Biggest Loser* has been broadcast in New Zealand, the UK, USA, Canada and the Middle East, and Adro has appeared as a special guest in the US series of *The Biggest Loser*.

Adro has been nominated for various national awards, including the prestigious Australian of the Year 2009, and is an ambassador for Workout World, Subway Australia, Avanti Fitness and HyperVibe whole body vibration. He is the founder and director of The New Me Weight Loss Retreat, certified personal trainer, life and weight loss coach and public and motivational speaker.

The New Me is his first book.

One of Australia's leading fitness and health writers, **Donna Jones** is a certified personal trainer, educator, journalist and author. She is the editor for her own series of magazines (including *Healthy Living* and *Slim Living*) and contributing fitness editor for major magazines (including *Australian Good Taste* and previously *Good Health & Medicine* and *The Sunday Telegraph's body + soul*). Her articles have also appeared in *The Sun-Herald, Cosmopolitan, Dolly, New Woman, She NZ, FAMOUS* and *Tony Ferguson Magazine*. An author in her own right, Donna has previously written three books on health, fitness and weight loss as the author of *Workouts for Everyone* (2005), and co-author of *If I Can, You Can – How I lost half my body weight* (2007) and *Winners Do What Losers Don't* (2008).

Acknowledgements

I would like to acknowledge everyone who has contributed to me being who I am today, in both positive and negative ways. I am who I am because of it. The journey is often just as important as the destination.

'He who gains victory over other men is strong; he who gains victory over himself is all powerful.' – Lao Tzu

The biggest events of my life that I feel have shaped me into the person I am today are fatherhood, *The Biggest Loser*, Camp Eden, having my skin surgery, and 'The New Me'. I'd like to acknowledge the people who were in my life during these moments but that would definitely take too long. To all these people, know that whatever experiences we had together – be it positive or negative – you are in my heart always for the impact you had on my life because you had something to teach me and I thank you for this.

I'm especially grateful to everyone who helped me find and grow into the person I am now; I am finally the person who I wish I had had in my life to influence me when I needed influencing the most.

To my family, I love and need you all, always and forever, and I can't wait until we are all able to sit back enjoying a thin, fit and healthy life together, well into old age.

Amanda Rix, darlin' if it wasn't for you I would never have even applied for *The Biggest Loser*, and so with Kris's groom suit as my dream outfit I went on to live your dream. Thank you for that.

Thank you to Crackerjack and the crew of *The Biggest Loser* because without you I wouldn't have had the opportunity to achieve all I have in life.

A big heartfelt thanks to Bob Harper and Jillian Michaels; I know that it was a job for you both, but for me it was a birth. I love you both forever. Not I, or anyone else, could ever have done for me what you two have.

Thank you to my fellow contestants, not only on my series but every *Biggest Loser* contestant. With what we have all been through I only wish and pray that you never need to go through it again. I wish you all the greatest of luck in love, life and happiness.

A big thanks to Grant Tomkins, you put yourself out so many times with your bulging discs in your back to make sure that I was up running every morning; regardless of the fact that it left you in bed for the rest of the day. I will appreciate that forever. Thanks also to Ray Kelly for your training and help in getting me over the line.

My gratitude to Jannah for allowing me to live in my now.

To all of my team at 'The New Me', without all of you guys we would not be able to spread our wings and fly as one. We have the right formula, the right people applying it and the right positive and life-changing environment; and we all have that because of who we are and what we bring.

To the team at Hachette, and Donna Jones, thank you for believing in my philosophy and bringing it to light through this book.

And lastly, I would really like to thank all of the people who I have met, inspired and helped since winning *The Biggest Loser*, and, of course, those of you reading this book; I don't think you will ever realise the impact you have had on my life. I am inspired daily to continue being all that I can be so that you have someone to look up to. I am honoured to be able to be that guy who gives you hope, and I will continue to keep growing forever.

Believe in yourself.

Adro

PART 1

The Old Me

The story of growing up (and out)

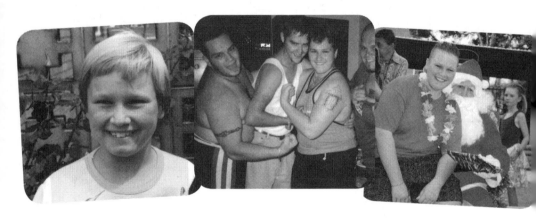

LEFT TO RIGHT: Me at 6 years old; That's me at 17 (third from the left) with my brother Damo, mate Matthew, and brother Mac, proudly showing off our Christmas tattoos; Me at 10 on Santa's knee. **OPPOSITE:** What a gorgeous bunch of boys we were, that's me (the baby and the blondie) at about 18 months, Damo and Mac.

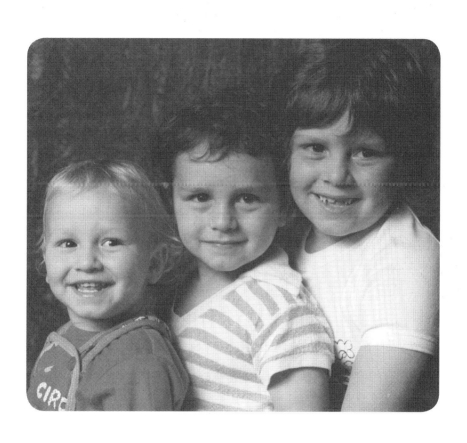

'There's always a story behind someone's
weight gain ... here's mine.'

Once upon a time there was a little boy who began to put on weight ...

Since I was a child I have always thought that it would be cool to write my own book, but it seemed like a fairy tale. What would I do that would be interesting enough to write a book about? Well, I did do something: I lost 52.3 kilograms (115.3 pounds) and became the first ever winner of the Australian series of **The Biggest Loser**. My fairy tale is more a fat tale but it still has a 'happily ever after' ending. I won my battle with the bulge, changed my life and did write my book after all. There's always a story behind someone's weight gain – nobody just becomes fat overnight – so let's start from the very beginning.

I was cute as a child, well, c'mon … blond hair and chocolate brown eyes … my mum thought so, anyway. I wasn't a big baby, nor was I chubby – at first. I was the middle child of seven children, the third son followed by a foster sister and three sisters, and growing up was fun, most of the time, but life in a big family had its challenges. I'm grateful for the experience and despite the shortcomings of my upbringing, I've always been a 'glass half full' kind of person by knowing that things could be much worse. That said, when people would ask me how many children I would like to have, I'd answer sarcastically, 'I'm one of seven children and I swear I will never be that cruel to anyone, let alone myself, again.' My mother and father separated when I was five. Dad moved out and I didn't get to see him much. Mum took over the role of both breadwinner and carer of the family. Life changed dramatically and looking back on this time in my life I can see that it impacted on my weight gain, as well as bad management of the food on my plate and my activity levels; I began life as the runt of the litter but badly managing my lifestyle and food choices changed me and my body shape.

Broken dreams *(Big changes can have big consequences)*

My parents splitting up not only affected me emotionally but it changed our standard of living. When they split up, Mum was about four months pregnant with my sister, Stephanie. So when she came along there were seven of us under the age of ten living in a three-bedroom house. We were a single-parent family, on the pension, Mum working part-time, with a mortgage. It was a massive job for my mother and she did brilliantly, I might add. I still admire her courage.

But this made everyday life pretty hard. Times were tough and Mum was on a tight budget. Because money was scarce our food had to be cheap, filling, versatile, plentiful and easy to prepare: enter carbohydrates. From very early on I became used to large serves of carbohydrates at every meal – plenty of pasta, bread and potatoes.

Mum was happy if our bellies were full (and so were we) and carbs fulfilled this role perfectly. You could feed the family dinner with three bags of pasta for a few dollars and some sauce, and know that they were full. And, if we ate meat and vegetables we were only able to afford cheap fatty chops or small amounts of vegetables so we filled up on bread rolls, because we were able to buy about eight rolls for a dollar at the local Vietnamese bakery. Basically, we were always eating either bread or pasta. I can still remember eating bread rolls with mashed potato and tomato sauce all the time – a double dosing of carbs! As you can see we were carb crazy; all loaded up with no place to go (except to my fat cells, it would turn out).

Over the years the carbohydrate habit stuck. I couldn't imagine living life without bread and pasta (pretty typical for an Italian, hey). But I later discovered it wasn't just the bread and pasta that caused my weight gain, it was the way I managed my meals too: each plate consisted of bread, pasta, potato or cereal when, instead, these complex carbohydrates (also called starches) should have been complemented with other healthy foods such as fruit and vegetables and lean meat (instead of taking up the whole plate!). You see the balance was way out and the scales were tipping over because they were stacked with too many starches.

Here was a normal day's menu:

Breakfast   *Bowl of cereal (usually sprinkled with extra sugar, against my mum's wishes!)*

Morning tea   *Muesli bar, crackers or potato chips*

Lunch   *Sandwiches or bread rolls or leftover pasta from the night before*

Afternoon tea *Sandwiches or bread roll*

Dinner   *Pasta or rice dish or a small amount of meat and vegetables usually with a big serve of bread or potato*

Dessert   *Not a common thing but when we did get a treat it was usually ice-cream, Madeira cake or Nutella on toast (for a chocolate treat)*

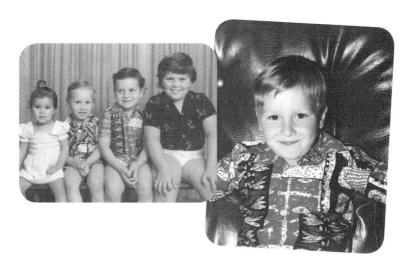

LEFT TO RIGHT: Ramona, me at 3 (love that shirt), Damo and Mac; Me at 4 (in another hot shirt).

WORKSHOP: Get the balance right
(on your plate and in your life)

Think back to your childhood. Do you remember significant events that might have triggered your emotional attachment to food?

Write down some key events and then the type of food you remember eating.

Your personal memories   *Your food memories*

1 2 3 4 5 6 7 8 9 10 11 12 13 1

Schoolyard nightmares *(Stay strong)*

I have many colourful memories of growing up in the neighbourhood of Auburn. But ultimately school was tough being an obese kid. Besides my brothers, I don't think there were any other fat kids in my primary school – it was the 1980s and the childhood obesity rate was nowhere near what it is today. If you struggled with your weight as a school kid, you too will have vivid and painful memories of being teased, just as I do. I can still remember the first time I was teased for being *the fat kid*. It was the time I went to school not realising that my shirt was inside out. It was an honest mistake and sounds harmless, but did I cop flak?

When I got to school that morning, as I was walking across the quadrangle, my teacher noticing my shirt, called out loudly across the playground, telling me to take more pride in my appearance and to put my shirt on the right way. With the whole class looking at me and already laughing I felt stupid and embarrassed (I pleaded with him to let me do it in the toilet block but he wouldn't let me). I had to take my shirt off and put it on the right way in front of my classmates. I could have died as they all laughed and pointed at me and my body. Some of them joked that boys weren't meant to have boobs. It was utterly devastating then and even now as I think about it. From then on the nicknames stuck – fatty boombah, fatty boomsticks, Fat Albert, the list is massive and it still hurts me to recall any more than these few. I seriously think the 'inside-out incident' had a massive impact on my life. At the time, I cried about it for days. It was definitely the beginning of me being the target of jokes and abuse for years to come.

WORKSHOP: Heal painful memories

Many overweight adults can recall specific moments of their childhood when they were humiliated or bullied because of their weight. This can leave real scars – on your self-esteem and the way you feel about your body, for life. Some people believe that these negative emotions can get stored in your body – literally locked inside your fat deposits – blocking you from reaching your goals such as losing weight and emotional freedom from always wanting to lose weight. If you think events in your past may be holding you back from reaching your true potential you need to talk about them with your friends or your family – or seek help with professionals, such as counsellors and psychologists. Even though it might be painful to revisit these moments, learning to deal with them can help unlock the key to some of your weight issues that are tied to your emotional state.

Try writing down some of your most humiliating 'fat kid' moments and see if you can write down what your response was then and now. By facing these issues as an adult and learning to move on, you can start working towards your emotional freedom (and more successful weight loss).

Embarrassing/negative childhood memories	Your response	Then	Now

Even though it might be painful to revisit past moments, learning to deal with them can help unlock the key to some of your weight issues that are tied to your emotional state.

Sitting on the bench *(Make sure you are active)*

Growing up, we never really played a lot of sports; Mum was definitely a little too worried about us playing rugby league or any contact sport for that matter. I guess at the time we didn't have too many other sports available and to most young boys in the western suburbs of Sydney it was rugby league or nothing. Remember it was the time of the greats like the Lamb boys and Sterlo and Fatty and Lyons. Rugby league was the in thing. But with no budding football career prospects I resigned myself to a youth of no exercise.

So thanks to inactivity and overeating (those carbohydrates again), when asked the question, 'How did you get fat?' my answer is 'bad management'.

WORKSHOP: Get active

How much does physical activity play a part in your life? Are you active for more than 30 minutes every day? Try keeping a record of your activity during an average week. Put in all the exercise you do, including any incidental activity such as climbing stairs rather than taking the lift, gardening, washing the car, walking to the shops. Once you can realistically see what you do each week you can then work on ways to up your activity level.

Monday ....

Tuesday ....

Wednesday ....

Thursday ....

Friday ....

Saturday ....

Sunday ....

Trapped inside a fat suit *(Rescue your self-image)*

I used to have a recurring childhood dream: I would be walking along one day and suddenly discover a zip on the side of my body and as I unzipped it I discovered that I wasn't really fat, that I had been trapped inside a fat suit the whole time and the thin me was there all along, desperate to step out. Each time I'd wake up, realise it was a dream, and feel trapped and angry. My anger came from hating the way I looked, suffering from what seemed like a tough childhood, and being the target of bullies and jokes. The more the kids picked on me and teased me, the angrier I got – not just at them, but at myself too. To make myself feel better I would eat more (more carbs). This just made me fatter and fatter, so those kids just picked on me even more, making me eat even more and so on and so on. *Read this again, a few more times, and a little faster each time, and then multiply that for every year between the ages of say six and 18 and you will begin to get an inkling of how I was feeling (and eating!) through all of it.*

Suppressed secrets *(Deal with painful, buried emotions)*

Life seemed tough in my younger years. As a single parent household, life for my mum must have been even tougher. As a family and as individuals, we were vulnerable. It's tough to write about this …

Through a social group my mother met a man. He seemed like a knight in shining armour – he was there for Mum and he wanted to help me conquer my weight. He regularly took me to the park, we'd run around, kick the ball, do some push-ups. I thought it was great and I began to feel hopeful that my dream of losing weight might come true. I could see a way out of obesity and the fat suit. I was rapt to be receiving this attention. But he was no hero, he became a little too interested in me and took advantage of my vulnerability. One day at the park, when no one was around he began to rub himself on me and touch me and make me touch him in places that I was sure had nothing to do with weight loss. It was utterly disgusting and this became part of a regular training routine.

I didn't tell anyone about the park, I buried the secret and carried this burden into adulthood, which has affected my life in ways I could never have known.

But how could I do anything? I thought. *If I say anything I might ruin Mum's happiness. I can't be responsible for that. This is all too much. I think I'll just be quiet. Maybe I can say I don't want to exercise anymore. Yeah, that will work. I'll just give up on wanting to change being fat and then I won't let him do what he is doing to me but my mum can still have what she needs and we will both be happy. I just won't train anymore and I'll just stay fat … maybe he won't like me if I get fatter and then he will only like my mum like he is meant to … yeah, he is meant to like her. She is great. Why does he like me anyway? I can't have this. I won't train and then I'll be okay and everyone will be okay!*

I'm sure that I had this conversation with myself for at least three months before I finally had the courage to stop training. I was so indescribably angry with this man. He told me he was able to help out by training me and this was to save me from being fat; he promised me that if I did what he said that he would be able to take away all of the life I didn't want. Instead, he took advantage of me and my family.

It was only a few months later, and my mum threw him out, after my sister complained about his inappropriate behaviour with her. Instead of doing what Nicole did, telling Mum and putting a stop to it, I took the cowardly option, not the courageous one like my sister, avoided him and convinced myself that I would be safer if I stayed fat, so he wouldn't like me anymore and would leave me alone. From then on, my weight became a shield – protecting me against abuse and unwanted attention.

WORKSHOP: Remove your shield

Many obese and overweight people hold on to their weight as a way of shielding themselves from something: unwanted attention; sexual or physical abuse suffered as a child; rejection; fear of failure by having an excuse to fall back on when things don't turn out in relationships, career and life; and not wanting to leave their comfort zone (because the familiar feels safe).

If you think you may be hiding behind your weight as a result of emotional issues, please raise these issues with a psychologist or counsellor. Holding onto secrets will only sabotage your weight loss efforts and your life. If this isn't an option, find a trusted friend you can talk to or get your feelings out by writing them in a daily journal or letter to someone (you don't have to send it).

During my childhood, I got counselling through a community organisation and my school. I went to counselling when my mum and dad separated, for being a fat kid, for being an angry kid suffering abuse. I wish I had taken those sessions more seriously, I may not have held on to so many issues!

To find an accredited psychologist in your state, contact the Australian Psychological Society (*www.psychology.org.au*). To find a counsellor, contact the Australian Counselling Association (*www.theaca.net.au*).

Obesity my fate? *(Get the right advice)*

The next big blow to add to my history of weight problems happened one day towards the end of primary school. All of us siblings were putting on weight, especially my oldest brother Mac (Mikele). This concerned my mother so she took him to see the doctor. When he came home he was upset and angry – so angry that he didn't want to talk about it with any of us. As the hours went by, we began fearing the worst for him. Then I overheard Mum on the phone saying that the doctor said that Mac had a hormone problem and would continue to get bigger and bigger, and that the rest of us kids would follow.

Whoa! Now slow down a minute … you mean to tell me that I'm stuck being not only this fat but fatter! Nnnnooo! This can't be real? Hormones? I thought only girls had hormone problems. That must be why I have boobs! I must be too much 'girl'!

I didn't quite understand it all but it left me feeling doomed. I cried upon hearing my fate. I don't even know if I was crying for me or for Mac or for all of us, as I'm sure that we were all having similar dreams of freedom; freedom from the torment that we were going through; freedom from a life trapped in a fat suit.

WORKSHOP: Find your weight excuses

Do you use your weight as an excuse to hide from the world or do you put off participating in certain social activities because you feel that your weight is a barrier to living your life to the full? Have a think about the 'weight excuses' you might come up with or have been told by doctors, family or friends. Once you have listed them, think about what's real and what's an excuse, or how relevant the excuses are.

Growing in size and anger *(Get the help you need)*

By the time I was ready to start high school, I had run away from home, come back, found God, lost God, and already started and stopped loads of diets. I tried many things to decrease my expanding waistline – everything from trying to eat less to following advice from aunties and uncles, friends and all sorts of people (who were also overweight but thought they knew so much better than I did, for some reason). I still remember my very first calorie-controlled diet that Mum put the whole family on. I still didn't lose weight so Mum took me to a doctor who immediately said, 'Boy, you're big!' He was right, of course, but no one wants to be told they're fat, especially not so bluntly. He then told me that I shouldn't let my weight go over the 75-kilogram (165 pound) mark and told me to eat mostly grains, fruit and vegetables, lean meat and fish and keep fats and sweets to a minimum – and to do some exercise every now and then. It sounded like a plan but it didn't really fit into the tight family budget that Mum was struggling to feed the family on. It just goes to show that your environment can have an impact on your weight. With the same poor eating habits my two brothers and four sisters, including my foster sister, all struggled with weight. This was way too hard to do on my own without any professional support and I struggled to control my weight gain.

Over the years, I went to see many doctors and they all started off by stating the obvious. 'You know you're obese', they'd all say. It was so frustrating. Of course I knew I was obese. I lived with me daily. I needed a better solution to suit my situation. My weight kept steadily increasing. By the time I was 10 years old, I was over 75 kilograms (165 pounds) and I was getting bigger and angrier.

Me against the world *(Find healthy ways to vent your anger)*

Things really went pear-shaped for me at high school. I was one of only a dozen fat kids at a school of 900 boys (and two of those were also my brothers!). There was a lot of anger through high school and my escalating anger made me a magnet for trouble. I looked for a fight as much as a fight looked for me. In class, I didn't pay attention, I was always late, talkative, stuffing around, sitting at the back of the room … just generally not wanting to be there. I even remember hitting a teacher with a one-metre ruler because he kind of brushed past and knocked me with it while trying to throw me out for being a pain. Even on the rare occasion where a special teacher would try and help me, I just pushed them away (as far away as those teachers who told me I was sloppy, fat and needed to take care of myself).

My second year of high school was no better: I was spiralling downwards and becoming self-destructive. The fighting was getting out of hand; you see at my school, if a fight started with one kid, by lunch-break you were not only up for a rematch with your original opponent, but five to ten of his cousins as well!

Parent–teacher interviews and detentions became common practice. Mum was constantly called up to the school to discuss my behaviour. It was truly me against the world.

Well, at least that was the way that it seemed. I felt trapped in a vicious cycle of destructive emotions – anger, hurt, hatred, fear and frustration – all stemming from the way I looked at myself and feeling frustrated about the way that the world looked at me. The world hated me and I hated it right back!

As my weight ballooned, my self-esteem deflated, and my anger and resentment gained momentum – all in direct proportion to one another it seemed. My inner hostility brewed to boiling point – from years of being bullied, coming from a broken home, suffering sexual abuse, the list went on. Combine all of this with a generous serving of self-hatred and the beginning of puberty (with all those crazy hormones) and you've got one cranky kid.

It took a parent–teacher night with a teacher telling me and Mum how much trouble I was, that I was a nuisance to so many other kids in the school, and, the clincher, that the teachers didn't see much in me and thought I would never amount to anything in life (boy, my already battered self-esteem really needed this!), to make me assess my anger.

WORKSHOP: Powerful self-esteem

Have you ever been told by a teacher, parent, boss, friend or partner that you're worthless? Well, I'm here to tell you that you are worth it. No matter where you've been, how many mistakes you've made and how many times you have tried to lose weight, you are worthy of a second, or third (or tenth!) chance and of having a better life – don't let anyone tell you anything different. How would you rate your self-esteem? List all the things that make you feel good about yourself. Then list all the things that you don't feel so good about. Have a good look at your list and see if you can turn some of the 'not so good' things around.

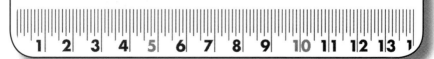

It doesn't matter how many times you get knocked down, what matters is how many times you get back up. Success is getting up one last time.

Glimmers of the new me (*Make that decision to change your life*)

Something happened to me that parent–teacher night; Mum and I cried all the way home in her Cortina stationwagon. Through her tears, Mum told me that she was trying to do the best she could to raise seven kids and that it wasn't right for me to be taking up too much of her time, energy and patience. If I didn't sort myself out, she told me, I would not be able to live with the rest of the family because they could no longer cope with me. When I got home that night I dragged my pathetic self to bed and told myself I was useless as I cried myself to sleep. Hitting this low point really made me stop and think about where I was headed.

I will never forget the way I felt when I woke up that next morning. Mum let me take the day off school and we talked. I told her I was sorry I had been so selfish and that I wanted to make myself count; I wanted to amount to something and not be a loser. I made a promise to myself that I would put effort into the parts of my life that I could control and I did. From that day, and the very next day, I went to school and I participated properly, I wore the right uniform, I went from sitting at the back of the class and being a goose to sitting at the front of the class and being a nerd! I wasn't going to let myself, or my mum down, and I wasn't going to be fat and dumb (as one of the teachers had called me). I consciously turned my out-of-control behaviour and life around. By the end of the year I was topping my classes (except physical education) and I was happier. I realised it was much more comfortable than being angry.

I realised that feeling angry and uncomfortable was a feeling that *I chose* and *I was choosing* to not feel it anymore. This change in attitude was the beginning of a new me, and what a difference to my life it made.

> *Choose your attitude, don't let your attitude choose you.*

I kept up my changed attitude into the next school year and, to my surprise, I was having a ball! I had a new outlook on life and I was in the top of my year for a lot of my classes – Mum was doing better also, and, life was good (except my weight still continued to climb). I no longer wanted to fight but my opponents still did. I had risen above it.

WORKSHOP: Change your bad behaviours

Think about parts of your behaviour or your life that you are not completely comfortable or happy with. Write them down in a list. Underneath each item you have written down, put into words what steps you can take to change that behaviour or that part of your life. Put these words into effect and write down how you feel each day in a journal. Keep a record of the change you feel is happening. Also make a note of how people are responding to you with your new positive attitude.

You can run, but you can't hide *(Face your demons)*

When I was about thirteen years old, my father came back into my life. During the course of my newfound father–son relationship, I had the opportunity to move in with my dad and stepmother, Dot. I didn't bother to stop and ask my mum what she thought about it at all and I think I really hurt her feelings. I think it was all said and done within a week, from idea to relocation, and I moved in a week after my fifteenth birthday. I was on my way to a new and wonderful lifestyle … or so it seemed.

It didn't take long for me to realise that the grass isn't always greener in another place and family. Have you ever been running through the house and not realised that the glass door was shut? Because it looked so good outside you ran right through the house until you hit the glass door. Well, my moving to the Central Coast was just like that. When you hit that glass door all of your expectations are shattered.

Moving to a new area meant starting at a new school. Of course things for me didn't really change. It was a co-ed school and I quickly learnt the meaning of 'better the devil you know' – turns out that the flak I got from the guys paled in comparison to the cruelty of the girls. My weight was still increasing and at my new school I endured the taunts and cruelty of the schoolyard again. I had learnt how to control my anger but I could not control the hurt I was now feeling. The negative thoughts about my weight quickly crept back into my head.

*Our attitude towards life
determines life's attitude towards us.*
– Earl Nightingale

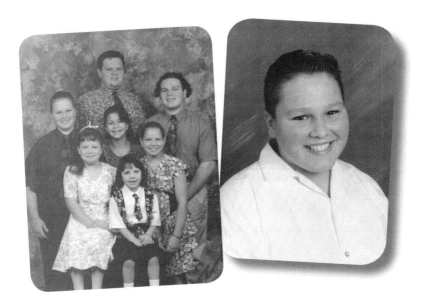

LEFT TO RIGHT: Official family photo with me (about 12 then), Mac, Damo, Mona, Stephanie, Nicole and Meryem; Me at 15 in the typical school photo, this was how I entered the life of co-ed schooling.

WORKSHOP: Reprogram your internal tapes

What repeating thoughts run through your mind like a broken record? What doubting self-talk do you constantly admonish yourself with? What you think, you create and what you believe, you manifest. Write down the negative internal dialogue that you find consuming your thoughts. Next to these thoughts write down a positive comeback and use these to interrupt the negative dialogue that you find yourself saying.

Negative thoughts   *Positive thoughts*

Girl stuff *(Dealing with hurt)*

One of the most upsetting times for me was in class one day when one of the cute girls stood up in front of everyone and sang a song to me, only this was no sweet serenade, it was the famous verse from Silverchair's song 'Tomorrow', with lyrics in the chorus referring to a fat boy. Of course, the whole class laughed at me. I don't even know if she got the words right, but the way she sang it will haunt me forever.

Now I found myself having to overcome a different emotion: hurt.

There's quite a big difference between walking around angry and walking around hurt. I found it much easier to control my anger, and the kind of hurt that you feel when you are being attacked or disappointed by the opposite sex – is a pretty tough break.

It wasn't long before food started calling for me again and the self-sabotaging talk (disguised as Mr Negativity) crept in: *It was just the guys, just Sydney, that was meant to be nasty and cruel. This is the new life, my new life, it was meant to be better. Why isn't it better? Why isn't it good? I know what I'll do, I'll go and eat, so that it will make me feel better and then if I get fatter that will give me more protection from all of the cruelties in the world and those nasty people will be blocked from the real me that's on the inside of this fat suit. My fat suit will keep me safe and then when I find the one or two people who I want to let inside, I will let them in because it will be my choice to let them in and I'll do it when I'm ready. Yeah, that's right, I am choosing to be fat now because it keeps the real me, the proper and sincere me, on the inside, hidden away for that special person who really chooses me for me. Then, I'll let the real me out and I will live happily ever after.*

What a head-case I was! People don't realise what goes on inside someone's head every day when they have to struggle with their weight; it's constant torment.

WORKSHOP: Overcoming your fears

Write down a list of things that you fear or hide from, such as facing a group, or standing up for yourself in a difficult situation. Next to your specific fears, write down positive ways to overcome these fears.

Giving up *(Hang in there)*

With the taunting and teasing back again, I didn't want to be at school anymore (again). But, despite this, I mustered the inner strength to keep striving for my dream of The New Me. I made a big decision.

At 15 and around 115 kilograms (253 pounds), I decided on New Year's Eve that I was going to cut out all the fats, oils, lollies, chocolate and all of that kind of crap. It was my first serious attempt at creating a better diet and lifestyle for myself.

I managed to keep up my resolution until around Easter that year (it's not what you're thinking) – turned out it was too much hassle for my dad and Dot to prepare separate meals. (Lots of families struggle with the logistics of managing and changing their mealtime culture and methods.) As it turned out I gave in, waved the white flag again, and returned to what was easy.

Some good did come of my reformed eating, however: even though I returned to eating everything the way I used to I was never able to eat butter or margarine again, not even something cooked with butter. I lost the taste for it.

WORKSHOP: You're always learning

Instead of feeling like a big fat failure every time you give up on a diet, and then running back to the cookie jar to soothe your pang of guilt for failing again, remember that you really never fail as long as you learn something and implement what you learn – even if all you learn is that the diet wasn't right for you, you still learn and you still gain. Make a list of your diets and weight loss attempts. Next to each one, write down something you learnt that can help you develop the right diet for you.

My attempted diet   *Lesson learnt*

1 2 3 4 5 6 7 8 9 10 11 12 13 1

Your goals are more important than just keeping the peace or satisfying someone else. It's not really putting people out as much as we feel it is and we are definitely not being difficult when trying to be healthy. Live life for you.

New beginnings *(You can turn your life around at any moment)*

It wasn't too hard falling back into my old fat ways. I spent most of Year 11 down at the local billiard hall as no one there made me feel bad or fat. Finally, by my sixteenth birthday, I'd had enough of school and being the fat kid. I'd organised a party and only three people showed up, out of the thirty or so I'd invited. My self-esteem was shattered. It was the straw that broke the fat boy's back – I couldn't handle it. I left school the week after, not because I didn't want to show my face, but more because running seemed like a good idea the first time and it seemed an even better idea the second time.

I wanted to leave the cruelty of adolescence behind, hoping that life as an adult (even a fat one) might be better; I guess it was time for me to grow up quick, or stick around and cop the abuse. I chose a new beginning.

Finding my way in the world *(Be true to yourself)*

At the age of 16 I'd left school and began working at a deli. Of course I sampled all of the wonderful food and my weight continued to escalate. I met a girl and we started seeing each other. I was in love and working and very happy. I didn't think about my weight at all. I moved on from the deli and started work in a jewellery store and loved it. After 12 months, I put myself through the trade, bought every book I could find on making jewellery and became a jeweller. For once in my life I felt as if I was in control, I was enjoying what I was doing and I felt great. But after four years I ended my relationship – I needed trust. I was heartbroken. My happy bubble burst and the negative thoughts came back to haunt me. At 20 I was around 120 kilograms (264 pounds). On the work front I took on a new hobby – building cars. To supplement my passion for cars I left the jewellery trade and took over a pizza shop at night so I could work on cars during the day. But as an adult with a busy career, now a new factor affected my weight – working long hours and not eating the right food. I had slipped back to my old food habits without even thinking about it. Again bad management of the various elements in my life took my increasing weight out of my control. I still struggled with low self-esteem even though I was becoming more successful in my business life. To hide my low self-worth I created an external bad-ass persona to keep people at arm's length. At 21, I shaved my head, as a way to empower myself. I continued to add to my tattoos and piercings, I guess I hoped people would fear me so I wouldn't have to let anyone in and risk getting hurt, again – and it worked.

Being anyone other than your true self will only cause you pain.

Getting serious about weight loss *(Tune in to your triggers)*

When I was 23 I met a girl named Sam. After two months together I let my guard down and invited her into my life – I asked her to marry me. And she said yes! About a month after we got engaged Sam became pregnant and we both made the commitment to give our child the life and opportunities that we never had as kids. When we found out she was pregnant I asked Sam if we could get married before the baby but she said no, because she didn't want to get married fat – no need to point out the irony here! I remember saying to her, 'Why not? I have to!'

My desire to become a more active father gave me the impetus to try to lose weight – again. I had tried to lose weight so many times – you name it, I tried it over the years: weight loss pills, shakes, fad diets. I would go through the standard protocol: join the gym and eat less which would work for me for the week or two that I did it. I would eat three Weet-Bix instead of six or eight, a salad sandwich or 'deli roll' from McDonald's instead of burgers, and used a cereal bowl, not a big dinner bowl, for my plate of pasta and made sure I didn't go back for seconds. I would manage to drop 5 kilograms (11 pounds) and no more, then I would give up. And this attempt was no different.

Several months in, Sam was holding the pregnancy very well – she was all belly – so she changed her mind and agreed to get married before the baby came. This was a big thing to me because I guess I'm a little old-fashioned in some respects. Our intimate wedding at our house was perfect; it was a day that was all about love and friendship; it summed up our relationship.

Despite many previous triggers to 'get serious' about needing to lose weight, there hadn't been one quite as shocking as when we went on holiday to the snow, just before the baby was born, and I had to be weighed to get my skis fitted properly. I jumped on the scales thinking I was around 125 kilograms (275 pounds). The reality – I was 144 kilograms (317 pounds). I nearly died.

On 11 October 2003 we had a baby girl: Odessa Jane Sarnelli. And from the moment I laid eyes on her, I knew that Odessa (named from the word odyssey) would change my life. Funnily 'odyssey' means a long and eventful or adventurous journey, and this is exactly the kind of journey I was about to embark on in my expedition of weight loss and personal transformation. And she, my beautiful baby girl, was going to be the reason I was to do it and the strength that got me through it.

WORKSHOP: Be your best for your kids

Your children offer a powerful motivation to do something about your weight. How many times have you been too tired to keep up with your kids? To run after them and revel in playtime? How often have you felt that your child might be embarrassed of the way you look, or, let down because you can't do the fun activities that other parents do. You may not be motivated to do it for yourself, but think of what your kids are missing out on because you're overweight. Not to mention how much they will miss you if you end up dead from obesity-related diseases. Write down a list of things you would really love to do with your kids and think of the small steps you can take to achieve these.

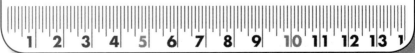

The wake-up call *(Listen to life's messages)*

Life certainly did change from that day on. I was the proudest dad in the whole world. I did as much as I could, falling short of breastfeeding Odessa (although I had the assets to do it, they just didn't work!).

Odessa was a great baby, and Sam and I were having an amazing time being parents. However, the one thing we did miss from our pre-parenting lives was spending time with each other. But I said to myself, 'If this is as lonely as it gets then it isn't so bad, I mean, after all, we have a beautiful baby girl.'

When Odessa was about four months old Sam decided that she wanted to go back to work so we searched around for a business that she could run. We set up a continental cake and coffee shop at Erina on the Central Coast. (No wonder I had a weight problem. The deli, the pizza shop, now a cake shop . . . I was setting myself up to be massive!) I must say when we had finished fitting it out it looked fantastic. And within seven days of trading we won an award for being one of the best businesses on the Central Coast.

When Sam decided that she was happier staying at home with Odessa I took it upon myself to run the coffee shop and the car business and was back to working 100-hour weeks. After eight months of running the coffee shop I awoke one night to a knock at the door at 3 a.m. only to learn that the coffee shop was up in flames. We lost the business completely and it was too expensive to try and recover our losses. After financially and emotionally surviving the coffee shop fire I expanded the panel shop and the business took on a new role as the NSW dealer for a company that made replica Hummers. With the combination of the loss of the business, emotional stress, increased workload and financial difficulties, my weight was once again inching upwards as I resorted to old habits.

It was only when Odessa was almost two that it hit home that my increasing size and lack of fitness prevented me from keeping up with a healthy, active toddler. This was my final wake-up call and I knew if I didn't do something now I would never ever be the father that I really wanted to be. I had to lose weight, once and for all.

WORKSHOP: Just do it!

Is your weight preventing you from doing the things you want to do? If you carried less weight what do you dream of doing? Write these dreams down and think of the ways you can make these dreams come true.

Achievements so far

Now it's your turn. At the end of every section of this book you have a chance to summarise where you are at. Set your goals, celebrate your achievements and stay on track with your own weight loss journey. With this part I hope you have:

✔ Identified events that have triggered your emotional attachment to food.

✔ Bravely faced down your worst fat moments and are on your way to emotional freedom (and successful weight loss).

✔ Discovered your personal level of physical activity and worked towards positive ways to increase this.

✔ Looked at your weight excuses and exploded your own self-myths.

✔ Rated your self-esteem and listed things that will make you feel better about yourself.

✔ Started a journal to keep a record of how you have consciously changed your behaviour and how people are responding to your new positive attitude.

✔ Turned the spotlight on your negative self-talk and found ways to interrupt any destructive mind chatter.

✔ Written down a list of your fears and thought of ways to overcome them.

✔ Listed all the diets you've been on and what you have learnt from them to help you create a diet that is right for you.

✔ Written a list of fun things you want to do for yourself and with your kids.

✔ Started the process of making your weight loss dreams and goals become a reality.

THE NEW ~~ME~~ YOU

Where are you up to?

WEEK: **WEIGHT:**

Emotional state

Physical state

Challenges

Accomplishments

POSITIVE PLUS:

I feel great today because

I am amazing because

I will/am succeed/ing because

GOALS:

INSPIRATIONAL QUOTE:

PART 2

Reality Meets TV
The journey from the old me to The New Me

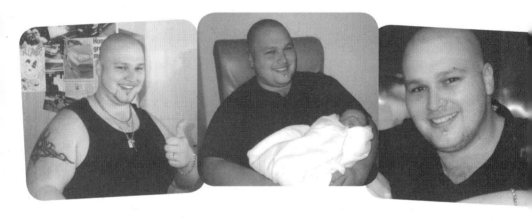

LEFT TO RIGHT: Me around the day I got married, weighing 150–155 kg; me holding Odessa when she was only minutes old – the proudest, most amazing moment of my life; me leaning over the counter at my continental cake and coffee bar. **OPPOSITE:** The glorious moment of winning *The Biggest Loser*.

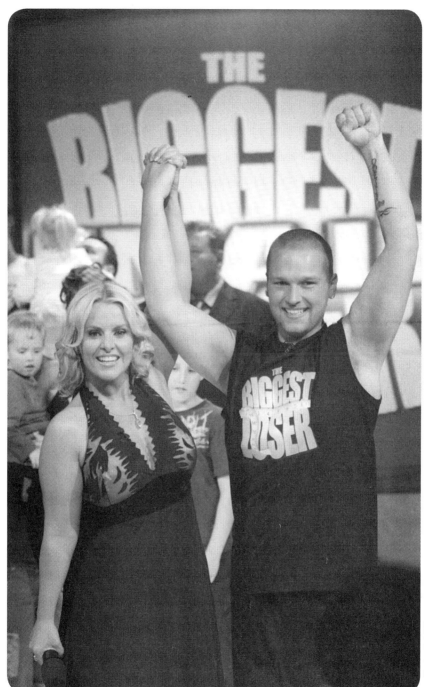

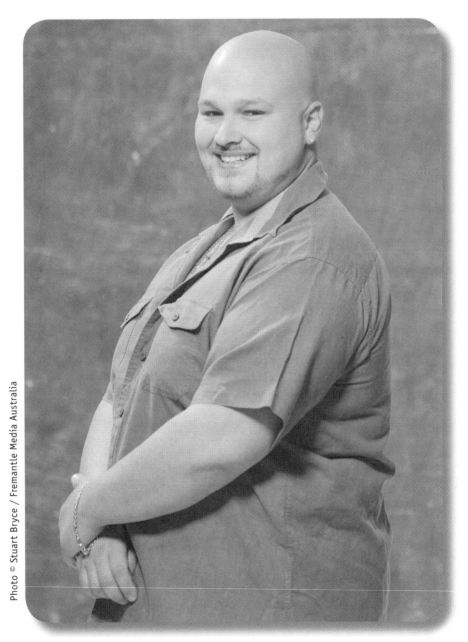

ABOVE: My final pose for *The Biggest Loser* promotions and the last photo of the old me (I would make sure of that).

*D*uring my time on *The Biggest Loser*, I dropped 51.3 kilograms (113 pounds) in 18 weeks. Of course, the number one question I get asked all the time is: How did you do it? On the night of the finale I promised that I was going to help as many overweight Australians beat obesity as I possibly could. Telling you how I did it is part of keeping my promise. My journey began with a decision ...

The decision to really make the weight loss happen this time felt all the more real with my daughter as the motive. Of course I went back to my usual weight loss routine thinking it would work again.

Einstein's theory of insanity: 'Doing the same thing over and over again and expecting a different result.'

According to Einstein I was clearly insane! For some reason, when it comes to dieting, you have a perpetual tendency to think that the reason you couldn't stick to the diet was because you failed, not because the diet failed you.

Within days of making my decision to change, I received a phone call from a friend of mine, who had got married earlier that year and I had been part of the bridal party. I felt really self-conscious about my weight at the wedding; not only did I have to wear a suit that didn't match the other groomsmen's because there wasn't one big enough and I had to have a different one made to fit my size, I was also on display in the church. I'm sure that most people didn't even notice, but I knew.

My friend was also struggling with her weight, and told me that she was going to apply for *The Biggest Loser* and thought that I should too.

My first reaction to her was to joke, 'Why? Do you think I'm fat?' After laughing, she explained to me that she thought that it could only be a good thing to have someone help you lose weight.

I had seen the American series and I knew how much weight they could potentially lose in a matter of weeks. The negative self-talk started: *No, there's no way that I would be able to do it. Even if I did lose weight I would never be able to lose that much that fast. I have been overweight my whole life, I wouldn't be able to just drop it so quickly, just like that! I can't be thin!*

My mind then switched to a safer possibility of being on the show: I thought that if I could just make it through to the audition stage I could mention that we built replica Hummers and we'd get a free plug on national television. Sounded like a genius idea. I decided that I would apply for the sake of the business (obviously I didn't believe in myself enough so I needed another reason to push me over the line). Plus it seemed easier to have an excuse ready if I failed to get on the program.

I spoke to Sam and it didn't take much convincing to get her on board.

> The greatest barrier to success
> is the fear of failure.
> – Sven Goran Eriksson

I downloaded the 16-page application form; they wanted to know about my whole life. I slipped back into my automatic 'everything-is-too-hard and I-won't-follow-through-with-it' mode that had haunted me my whole life. Even today, I still catch myself wanting to slip into this mode, although I am a bit more disciplined with it now as I try to be more aware of it. I decided to get Sam to fill in the forms for me. It was Sam's support and her words that forced me to post the form:

You keep on going on about how you wish you could get things done and you have an opportunity to do just that and you're not even going to bother doing it? Just do it, Adro!

And with this drop of the envelope I decided that I was going to be open to whatever came my way and follow through with my goals, which I didn't have a good track record with. (See, positive changes were already happening.)

It's funny how easy you quit, when you're a quitter.

I know that sounds stupid but it's true; it doesn't take much at all to give up when that's what you're used to doing. I used to hate giving up but, boy, I was good at it.

I suddenly realised that there was a possibility that I could be a part of *The Biggest Loser.* I felt a bit nervous and a bit excited but the cool thing was that I felt okay with the possibility. I set myself a goal of reaching 110 kilograms (242 pounds) with an absolute dream, most-likely-in-another-lifetime, goal of 100 kilograms (220 pounds). I noticed that I was already starting to think positively.

Two weeks later I received a call letting me know that I'd made it through to the auditions of *The Biggest Loser.* Telling Sam and the boys at work was pretty exciting. I couldn't believe that I'd made it, even though Sam said she had always believed I would make it.

WORKSHOP: Follow through with your goals

In the journal you began in Part 1, write down a list of positive thoughts about your life, about doing an activity or completing a task that seems way too hard. Resist the urge to put this off and really go for it. Next to this list, write down the outcomes that occur when you consciously change your mindset.

Positive thoughts   *Outcomes*

| 1 | 2 | 3 | 4 | 5 | 6 | 7 | 8 | 9 | 10 | 11 | 12 | 13 |

Auditions *(Be open to possibilities)*

The day of the audition arrived. I walked into the room with the other potential contestants and my first thought was that I was really underdressed as I was in casual clothes. Everyone else was dressed up for the occasion. Despite this, for the first time in my life, I actually walked into the room without using my usual protective behaviours: slouching, dropping my shoulders, avoiding eye contact, dragging my feet, pulling my shirt outwards away from my stomach and hiding up the back of the room with big people to find safety in numbers. This was really liberating and I suddenly realised how much my self-esteem had been affected by my weight issues. It brought me to my knees to realise how uncomfortable I was in my real life.

'Hi, I'm Adriano,' I said with my head held high. 'Sorry I'm late, I got lost. Does anyone know if I'll get a ticket for parking my (replica) Hummer out the front?' *Great, got that plug in already.*

Each person had their turn at introducing themselves. What was I going to say?

My moment arrived. I stood up and introduced myself. I thought about standing up and saying, 'Hi guys, I'm Adriano, and I'm an alcoholic', but sensed this was no time for my usual jokes. In the first few minutes of my introduction, I managed to mention a few times that I had a shop that made those replicas. *God, I hope they use these audition tapes. I wonder how many more times I can plug my business?* At the end of my introduction I said, 'And I don't know what I'm giving permission for but everyone else has given theirs so I will, too.' Most of the guys laughed, but I'm sure that there were a few people in there also thinking that this jerk wasn't even taking this seriously.

The producers then explained that what I was giving permission for was a privacy agreement for them to be allowed to use the footage and whatever we did today in the making of the TV show, which would be shown to other people.

The next thing we had to do was what they called 'speed dating'. We had to speak to someone about ourselves for one minute and then listen to the other person speak about themselves for another minute. We did this five times and were asked to share some of the things we learnt with the group. Thankfully, I took in enough to pass the test!

After our speed dating session, we were informed that some of us were going home and others would be staying on for a one-on-one interview. They congratulated everyone on getting this far from the 6600 people who had applied for the show.

When I heard my name called out I didn't listen well enough to know if that meant I was staying or going. Then another guy told me that I had made it through to the next stage! I could hardly believe it, because those things just didn't happen to me, ever!

As we waited for our turn to be interviewed, we (there were about ten of us shortlisted from Sydney, plus more from elsewhere around the country), started talking about the slogans or phrases for the shirts we would wear if we got through. I was the only one who thought maybe a joke could be what they were after and started tossing some funny slogans around: 'Wide load'. 'Caution: Vehicles backing up'.

I was in no rush to get home as I was really enjoying being so comfortable around these people. Wasn't that weird? My whole family and most of my friends were big but I had never been this comfortable around a bunch of strangers. On the other hand, the fact that I felt so comfortable with these people was disturbing because I never felt this way around healthy weight people; I didn't want to spend the rest of my life only feeling comfortable if I was around big people.

My one-to-one meeting was like an interrogation minus the light shining in my eyes. There was a panel of producers and a guy ready to video the interview.

I was asked to share some information about myself, including how much I weighed and why I wanted to lose weight. I told them I sat at around 135–140 kilograms (297–308 pounds) and my main reasons for wanting to lose weight were my beautiful girl, my wife and a business I would like to keep building. I admitted that I would love for my wife to be able to enjoy being with me as much as I enjoy being with her. I also explained a little about the early history of my childhood weight gain and how I went through school being the fat kid.

They then asked me what my goal weight was, and I readjusted my perhaps-in-another-lifetime goal of 100 kilograms (220 pounds) to 95 kilograms (209 pounds) because I felt under pressure to impress them with the possibility of such a big weight loss. However, I didn't really believe in my heart that that was an achievable goal for me.

After some more intense questions I came to another realisation that I was constantly putting up sabotaging thoughts and actions to avoid really getting down to why I was overweight, how I was going to lose weight and why it was important to me.

WORKSHOP: Believe in yourself

Do you really believe you can lose weight? Of course, your initial reaction is most likely yes, but if you sit with yourself quietly for a few moments, and look deep into your heart, do you really believe you can lose the weight and have the body you long for?

Perhaps family, school bullies, doctors or even friends have dented your self-belief. If you don't believe you can achieve, that's okay, you don't have to in order to get started, but sooner or later you will have to find that belief in yourself if you are to truly make your dreams come true. Start thinking about what you want to achieve and start believing that you can do this. Write these thoughts down in your journal like a mantra and repeat this to yourself daily.

The journey begins *(The journey of 1000 miles begins with one step – Chinese proverb)*

I told every single person that I ran into and spoke with that I might be on *The Biggest Loser*. My level of excitement was so high that everyone I met was affected by it. I found myself doing something unfamiliar: making positive affirmations, instead of letting Mr Negativity take control. I affirmed to myself: *I can and will do this*. I also committed to continuing with my own weight loss regardless of whether I made it onto the show.

I received a phone call from the production company telling me I was in the final 24 and I had to have a medical assessment and then a psychological assessment.

Then, on Thursday, 1 December 2005, I received another phone call from the production company and after a few more questions was told those three words that I was dying to hear: I was in!

At first, I couldn't tell anyone, including my family, because they wanted to capture their genuine look of surprise on camera. Needless to say, this was no easy task. I wanted to tell everyone.

There were a couple of days of pre-filming, where they took some 'a-day-in-the-life-of-Adro' type footage.

They then asked me to strip down to my underwear and nominate on my body all of the things I hated about it; it was what they called 'body mapping'. This was something that was pretty tough for anyone who struggles with their weight, for anyone for that matter! I had to stand there and identify to the camera what I didn't like about my fat, sloppy body. My first reaction was to make a joke about it: 'Could I tell you what I like about it? It would be a whole lot faster.'

But a joke wasn't going to let me off the hook, so I started: 'I don't like my boobs, well they shouldn't be there at all; I hate the fact that I have bigger boobs than any male I have ever met and a lot of females too; I hate my belly and apron and the fact that it hangs over so far; I hate my arms, they are so big and floppy and they drive me insane.' And then, turning around with my back facing the camera I said, 'What about this? I have more rolls than a bakery back here and the whole thing is disgusting!'

It didn't take long for me to relax and just continue to put my body down. I hated being fat and there was no point in hiding it, especially hiding it from myself. I made a conscious decision that this was really *it*; this was to be the last time I was going to have to lose weight because I was going to lose it for good!

The time came to say goodbye to Sam and my little girl, and it was off to stay in a hotel in Sydney for a few days to do some pre-filming and photo shoots for promotional material.

One of my favourite promotional shots involved me jumping into a pool telling the camera that I wanted to be around to see my daughter get married and no longer be a back-bench father. These messages were really important to me because they were the reasons I was willing to give up my life as I knew it to lose weight and give myself a shot at being all that I could be.

Finally, the big day arrived: 5.30 a.m. Monday was our wake-up call to get picked up and make our way to the house, in Sydney's northern suburbs, where the show would take place and lives would change. As we were driven across the Sydney Harbour Bridge I said to myself: 'Let's change my world.'

What are you willing to sacrifice in your life to make the changes you need?

WORKSHOP: Body mapping

Strip down to your underwear and stand in front of a mirror. Have a go at 'body mapping'. List all the things that you don't like about your body and acknowledge what you see honestly. Then make the commitment to do something about it for good.

What I don't like about my body

The diary *(Your life and weight can change in a matter of months)*

For those of you not familiar with *The Biggest Loser*, there is a red and a blue team and each team competes for the most weight loss each week. At the weekly weigh-in, all the contestants are weighed and our individual weight loss goes towards the total weight lost by each team; the team with the least overall weight loss faces elimination, the biggest loser from the losing team is safe, while the rest of the team is up for elimination. The losing team then votes for the person they want to be eliminated from their team. The one with the most votes gets eliminated and sent home.

The red team, to be trained by Jillian Michaels, consisted of myself, David Hylander, Josephine 'Jo' Cowling, Kristie Dignam, Shane Giles and Ruth Almeida de Campos.

The blue team, to be trained by Bob Harper, consisted of Catherine 'Cat' White, Arthur 'Artie' Rocke, Harry Kantzidis, Fiona 'Fe' Falkiner, Tracy Moores and Vladimir 'Big Wal' Milberg.

My starting weight was 136.5 kilograms (300 pounds). I had already lost some weight before the show on my own weight loss plan when I decided to finally do something about my weight.

We entered the 'White House' which was to be our home for the next ten weeks. It was set up to enable us to fend for ourselves and we weren't allowed to make contact with the outside world.

The food in the kitchen was far healthier than any of us was used to and the first rude fact that I learnt during The Biggest Loser *was that food isn't there to please the tongue* (I know, I couldn't believe it either), *only to fuel our bodies.*

We met our trainers, Bob Harper and Jillian Michaels, the next day as they ran up the driveway. It was pretty exciting to see the two people we had been watching on the American version of The Biggest Loser *rock on up.*

On greeting us, something Bob said really resonated with me.

> You need to believe in yourself, we cannot and will not do this for you, we can show you how, teach you and be your tools but we cannot and will not be able to do this for you; you have to do it for yourself, want this for yourself and believe in yourself.
>
> – Bob Harper

Upon hearing these words, I realised I had to take ownership of my weight problem. This is a philosophy I now live by and teach others to this day. Something about these words made me want this for myself, not just for my daughter.

> Only you can lose the weight, and you alone – everything and everyone else you encounter on your weight loss journey is merely a tool to facilitate your **own** weight loss.

My life on The Biggest Loser *had begun.*

Week 1

Our very first training session was on day two and it was hard! It was mainly a cross-training session using the cardio gear, such as the treadmills and cross trainers, combined with exercises on the floor where Jillian had us do a whole lot of body weight exercises, such as squats, lunges, push-ups, mountain climbers (you can find these exercises in Part 4 in the 'Move More' section) and loads of other exercises I had never even heard of, let alone done before. I remember thinking, 'My god, how much longer can this go for? Can it get any harder?' It did get harder, but somehow I made it through the session. It was very full on and I kept thinking that I didn't like Jillian anymore.

The first week was all about testing my body, mind, emotions and patience. Although I was cheeky the whole way through the first week and Jillian was always punishing me with extra exercises, I think that I wanted this in a way, because every time I stopped for a breath I beat myself up thinking that I wanted to go further, harder, faster. I was able to pull through and push myself. My personal motto for the first week was 'Just keep on keeping on'.

We lost the first week's weigh-in; an injury made David an easy out for the other team members and they chose him to be eliminated. In the short time I had known him, I had grown quite fond of David; we connected from the first moment and he felt like a brother. Unfortunately my strong attachment to David wasn't enough to see him stay for longer than the first week. Sadly, I bid goodbye and wished the best of luck to my newfound friend.

I lost 7.7 kilograms (17 pounds).

Week 2

The second week saw the exercise routines stepped up a notch in a bid by Jillian to save the red team from going through another elimination. I was learning a lot about my body by this stage: that it was able to do (even reluctantly) what Jillian and I told it to do and I felt that I was able to train harder than anyone else in the red team, which gave me a sense of achievement. Week 2 was the week over Christmas and I really struggled with being away from my family, so focusing on my training was a good distraction.

We had to cook and organise our food, so it didn't take long to get into the rhythm of eating better. Jillian advocated freedom of food choice. She told us to stick to a set calorie amount and that we could enjoy the freedom so long as we stuck to our calorie quota. Without the distractions from the outside world we were able to completely focus on the major weight loss principles: healthy food and regular exercise.

We lost the second week's weigh-in again, and the elimination saw Ruth and Kristie portrayed as double-crossing Jo to keep me from going home. Right from the start Kristie, Ruth and I had envisioned ourselves making it to the end, as we had met at auditions and were friends from the beginning. We all voted for Jo and she was sent home. With Jo's going home this week, the red team's morale was slipping because we had not won a major challenge yet and we were two team members down.

I lost 2.4 kilograms (5 pounds).

Week 3

It was time for the red team to make a change and a difference in the game. The week's challenge saw me play an absolutely brilliant game of soccer with former Sydney Football Club star, Dwight Yorke. What a guy and what an absolutely amazing game – everything was surreal about it, from a fat guy playing soccer at Aussie stadium, where the greats play sports, right through to how it felt to not only score all of the four goals that the red team won by, but also to see how excited Dwight was getting as I played the game. I did the greatest palle kick (named after freestyle soccer star, Rickard 'Palle' Sjolander; a kick where you get under the ball as it's in the air and jump up into an almost back flip to kick the ball back up over your head) the world had ever seen. I nearly died, Dwight nearly died, and once it aired, I think the rest of Australia nearly died! It was the most fun I had ever had and I felt like the king of the world; that day I could have been David Beckham, Michael Jackson, Brad Pitt, Tom Cruise ... anyone I wanted to be.

Winning this game gave me a trophy, a giant world cup trophy labelled 'Losers World Cup', which is one of my most prized possessions. It also gave the red team the chance to bring Wal, from the blue team, across to our team.

With the loss of the blue team's strongest contender this week's weigh-in saw a win for the red team. The blue team sent Cat home. A real shame as Cat was big and beautiful and reminded me of one of my sisters.

I lost 1.8 kilograms (4 pounds).

Week 4

The fourth week was another powerful week for the red team. Although Wal had to sit out of almost every challenge, the red team's morale was up and we were not going to fool around this week.

I had a great week of training. Jillian was training Wal and myself on the floor together, because I could keep up with him, and I remember feeling that I could take on the world. I was growing stronger and more confident and, for the first time in my life, started to enjoy exercise!

We saw the blue team lose in the weigh-in and face elimination. Without using many brain cells, the blue team sent home one of the strongest contenders, Harry. This was exactly what we needed.

My weight, on the other hand, wasn't exactly doing what it was meant to do. I was supposed to be losing more weight and be rewarded more than I was for my hard training efforts. I was also eating under my calorie allowance. Jillian was getting a little frustrated with me and I began to get frustrated with her; I needed someone to blame. Nonetheless, I continued to push on and the tension between Jillian and I continued to grow.

I lost 2 kilograms (4.4 pounds).

Week 5

The game took a turn that saw us split into pairs with me matched up with Ruth. We weren't too happy, as we both believed that it would be the ruin of us because we were both poor performers when it came to the scales.

Ruth and I found ourselves up for elimination, along with Tracy and Artie who lost the week's challenge and received a 2-kilogram (4.4-pound) penalty as a consequence.

Fe (Fiona) voted for Ruth and I to go and for Tracy and Artie to stay, but the other team members felt Tracy and Artie had outstayed their welcome and without them the rest of us felt there would be less conflict in the house.

With my rate of weight loss still not making a dent on the scales, I was now really frustrated. I argued with Jillian about why I was struggling with my weight, which left our relationship a little sour come the start of the following week.

I lost 0.6 of a kilogram (1.32 pounds).

Week 6

This week, our groups of two were split up and it was every man for themselves. No more red and blue; we all wore individual colours. I thought this would be the point where I went home; I wasn't losing enough weight, and to not have a team with me to keep me afloat I figured left me without a chance.

Despite my repeated attempts to get to the bottom of my less than impressive weight loss, I felt that Jillian wasn't listening to me.

A chance came up to gain immunity at the week's weigh-in so you couldn't be up for elimination – the catch was you had to eat cupcakes and find the winning one that granted immunity. You didn't have to take part; it was your risk and your risk only to consume that many excess calories and possibly undo your weight loss if you didn't win the game.

Choosing to take part in the immunity game led to a big fight with Jillian as she always told us not to go for immunity. By the end of the fight Jillian no longer wanted to train me and I no longer wanted to train with her. I decided I would rather throw it all away and head home than train with her again.

Bob stepped in and I began training with him and this was the beginning of my huge weight loss. I responded better to Bob's more passive approach (or maybe it was, as Jillian pointed out, having the older male figure fill my absent father figure issues). I felt like I had someone who loved me and genuinely wanted to help me and me to help myself. Bob also changed my diet from the freedom of food choice to a high protein/no- or low-carbohydrate way of eating. I modified Bob's advice and developed an eating pattern, which I still follow today: low fat, low carb, low calorie, high protein. All combined with the freedom of choice.

My change in attitude and diet sparked the beginning of me making my mark, recording a huge weight loss this week, beating everyone except Fiona, and defeating Wal – this triumph sent who we all considered the fiercest competitor home. This still didn't leave me looking like much of a threat to the other competitors; secretly, though, I felt that my only challenger was Shane.

I lost 7.7 kilograms (17 pounds).

Week 7

I wanted to maintain my weight loss momentum. I had my head down and my bum up as I worked hard to stay in the competition. I was up alone every morning on the stepper, burning calories at a rate of 150 per 10 minutes. I was training more hours than anyone else. I knew what I wanted and I could see my potential. I was in control. As for my self-belief, it was right up there, probably the best it had ever been.

In the weigh-in, Ruth and Fiona fell below and were up for elimination. As Ruth, Kristie and I had agreed to keep to the original plan of sticking together, I prepared myself for Fe's departure, voting for her to leave. But, Kristie voted differently and sent Ruth on her way. It was at this point that I knew I could no longer trust anyone and had to really make sure that I made every second count.

I lost 2.4 kilograms (5.28 pounds).

Week 8

This week turned out to be a major turning point in my life. Kristie, Fiona, Shane and myself headed up to Camp Eden, on Queensland's Gold Coast in Currumbin Valley. During my stay I truly found myself and I realised that a new beginning was on the horizon – all I had to do was embrace my self-discovery and let my spirit shine through. I realised that I had the control, power and ability to be who and what I wanted to be in my life rather than settling for who or what I was just because I felt I couldn't do or be anything more than that. This happened as a result of doing the Braveheart challenge: a jump from a 65-metre tall tree wearing just a harness. Conquering this challenge made me realise that there was a lot more to this weight loss thing than just shedding a few kilos, and that I had fooled myself by thinking the reason I was overweight was because I had a time problem and not a weight problem. Being confronted by a fear of heights and achieving something I had never done before in my life was amazing. This spiritual shift had a colossal effect on my life. Me diving off the platform was The New Me. For the first time in my life I felt free.

Once we returned home from Camp Eden, we weighed in and I had defeated the only real contender left in my mind, Shane – not only for the first time, but for the first time that it really counted, which saw me, Kristie and Fe as the final three.

I lost 3.6 kilograms (8 pounds).

My Eden epiphany

On the platform, 65 metres up, looking out across the valley I had my epiphany, for it was atop that tree that I came to the realisation that I was not obese just because of what I ate and what exercise I didn't do; I realised that I was obese due to issues I was holding onto.

Simply climbing to the top was scary enough; I've always been afraid of heights. Reluctantly, I made the climb and realised what a big mistake I had made. I was so frightened I had to hold back my tears.

As I turned around and slowly shuffled to the edge of the tiny platform I suddenly started having visions. My whole life (as a fat person) flashed before my eyes – all the teasing and taunting, heartache and unhappiness. I saw pictures of my childhood, buried images of being abused, flashes of growing up fighting with my brothers and sisters, images of my mum and dad together and separated, fights I was in through my school years, the way I felt when I moved away from my all boys' school and went to a co-ed school and how hard it was to not only have boys harass me but girls also, I saw my brother who I hadn't spoken to for a couple of years after a fight we had, I felt the sting of past girlfriends, right up to my present life and the angelic image of my daughter. I saw so many things as I stood there motionless, awash with a swirl of uncontrollable emotions. It was almost like I was ticking off and acknowledging everything that had happened to me in my life, that had contributed to the person I was today, the person standing up on that platform, preparing to jump.

Somehow the visions and overwhelming feelings stopped and I felt ready to jump; to let go and release everything that had happened to me in my life that made me who I was. I began chanting the words: 'The New Me, The New Me, The New Me', and I spread my arms out like butterfly wings and let go.

Bob had been screaming words of encouragement for the whole 28 minutes I was up there, but now all I could hear was the sound of the trees. As I left the platform I felt myself leave my body; I was floating out into the crisp air, watching my body falling off the edge, splitting into two separate bodies. It was the most remarkable thing I have ever experienced. The old me – fat and sad, confused and scared – remained on the platform, helplessly trying to grab hold of the figure leaving the platform. The fat figure became a shadow, grey and lifeless, as the figure leaving the platform became brighter. It was this brighter figure that I found myself in again when I made it to the ground.

I was so overwhelmed by what I had just experienced that I was crying helplessly. I hugged Bob as I was so emotional and couldn't believe what I had just been through. With my feet planted firmly on the ground, I turned to look back up to the platform and I could still see the shadowy figure of my former self, stuck and scared. At that moment I knew that I was never going to be overweight or obese again; I knew that whatever it was that I needed to acknowledge, accept and let go of in order to truly be free and be me I had done.

This spiritual shift had a colossal effect on my life. When I look back, I realise that the figure that left the platform was a figure of me today: the thin Adro, 'The New Me'. For the first time in my life I felt free.

Week 9

In true TV style they decided to bring the contestants back for a wild-card entry, which would allow one successful contestant to stay. We all knew that this would be Shane, Wal or Harry and we didn't want a part of it. Feeling cheated by the new game plan we decided to make a pact and do what we could to see the intruder sent on their way.

In response to this, Mr Negativity invited himself back in to my headspace, and he was laughing louder than ever. He kept yelling in my ear, 'I told you so' as the invited contestants returned to line up on the driveway. As a result, I started thinking that I wasn't worthy of something like this. What an idiot I was to think I had defeated Mr Negativity. What a cruel world to play such a game on me. I knew I wouldn't win. What a waste of time. I kept thinking I'll be the same 'fat jerk' that I've always been!

We were meant to finish the show and go home this week, but two weeks earlier the producers asked us if we could extend our stay for an extra two weeks and we agreed as we all thought it would be a good way to ensure that we had an extra two weeks worth of weight loss. (We never expected them to fill the two weeks with this.)

We didn't weigh in this week; only the returning contestants did as they vied for a place back in the competition.

Week 10

Week 10 was tough – mentally, emotionally and physically. Harry was the one to make it in as the wild card entrant and I didn't know if I would be able to beat one of the big boys again. I was fearful about how I was going to keep my place in the final, but I didn't have a choice – it was happening and I had to accept it. I had to give more than my everything. I trained harder, I dieted harder, I thought harder, I prayed harder, I dreamed harder.

The emotional torment that I was going through was full on, I felt that everything I had worked so hard for was about to fall apart, to be taken away from me, and I felt powerless once more. Being so close to the end and having a win in sight, I lost focus of the weight loss for a moment and began to only see the game.

I lost a lot of weight, but fell short (within a kilo, almost 2 pounds) of being able to send Harry home and carry on with my team mates. It was a very emotional time from the moment I was on the scales to the moment I was eliminated in the elimination room. It took all of my strength to not revert back to the old me, that angry guy in Years 7 and 8. Instead, I thanked the host, A.J. Rochester, for the experience, shook her hand and walked away. I wanted to punch something in the elimination room but I didn't – I did punch the concrete wall in my room as I packed up, though, and then broke down!

I lost 6.5 kilograms (14.3 pounds).

Week 11

This was training at home for seven weeks before the finale. I decided when I was eliminated that I was going to be the biggest loser, even if I couldn't win it, by still losing the most weight. I was going to fight for what I believed was going to be the biggest 'Up yours!' as I imagined myself returning with the greatest weight loss of all the contestants. I was going to prove to them that they had made a mistake by voting me off over a wild card entry. I got in contact with a personal trainer, Ray Kelly, to help me do this.

On leaving the house, I was hit with some major bombshells, which seriously tested my commitment to not give up. While I had been away my business had dwindled without my help.

And I discovered how much of an impact my being away had had on my family: Odessa was absolutely covered in eczema due to the stress of not having her father around; Sam was an emotional wreck from having to deal with the business and becoming a single parent when she needed me there.

To top things off, I left the house weighing 102.3 kilograms (225.06 pounds) and then within the week, put on 10 kilograms (22 pounds), while I was laid up in hospital as a result of needing surgery on my hand from slipping over while cleaning out my workshop. Despite these setbacks that made me feel like going back into my shell I somehow managed to dig into whatever inner-strength reserves I had left, and instead of reverting back to the old me, I chose to use everything that was happening around me to build strength from As the saying goes: 'That which doesn't kill you, only makes you stronger.'

Several weeks into training at home (I even trained with my bloodied hand in a sling, I was that determined), I did receive a little boost that lifted my spirits. To my surprise A.J. came a knockin' on my door. First, she couldn't believe how much extra weight I had lost and how much I had changed. She then told me that I was back in the running for a shot at the title of The Biggest Loser! Jillian had campaigned to get me back in the final because she didn't think it was fair that Harry was allowed back in.

In seven weeks I lost 27 kilograms (59.4 pounds).

Victory (Sweat + sacrifice = success– Charlie Finley)

Week 12

I had trained for the last four months for this day. Making it all count today was the focus of the last seven weeks of training at home, as well as all the struggles and pain I had put myself through.

We had a behind-the-scenes weigh-in the day before, and although we didn't get to see our weight, I had a feeling that I had won. I remember thinking how I was never, regardless of the outcome at the finale, going to go back to my old ways. I was going to go on and continue this journey forever.

At the finale Harry got up and weighed 112.7 kilograms (247.94 pounds), a loss of 37 per cent of his total body weight; Kristie weighed in at 66.1 kilograms (145.42 pounds), a loss of 36.93 per cent total body weight; and we all knew Fiona was never going to be a threat. I was pretty confident I had the win in the bag.

I stepped onto the scales. Although I battled with negative self-talk, I still visualised my moment of triumph time and time again. The scales clicked and everyone went silent … 85.2 kilograms (187.44 pounds), a loss of 37.8 per cent of my total body weight. I had won by less than one per cent! Just a couple of hundred grams determined my fate! (In the end, I believe I won by the weight that had been lifted off my shoulders; the burden of a lifetime of obesity).

The room was silent, the only sound I heard was my brother Mac's scream and I knew that I had done it. The feeling was truly indescribable and whenever I go over this event in my mind I still get butterflies in my stomach and sweaty palms. It was one of the most extreme moments of my life.

That night after beating my own obesity demons, I made a promise to help as many overweight Australians beat obesity as I possibly could; I was going to pay my opportunity back.

I lost 51.3 kilograms (112.86 pounds) during my journey on The Biggest Loser.

Taking out *The Biggest Loser* marked the beginning of a new life as a thin and healthy person. It meant that I had set myself a personal goal, and followed it through with determination and a fire that I had never thought was in me.

Winning my weight loss war was the proudest victory of my life. It elevated my emotional and mental state and opened the door to a new way of living. For the first time in 20-odd years I started to live. I discovered the difference between just being alive and living life. Finally, I was able to scream from the top of the world, 'I choose life'!

Back to reality *(From the old me to The New Me)*

Having the energy to play with my daughter was just one of the amazing new things I could do that I previously couldn't because my weight held me back. On my first play outing with Odessa we had so much fun that she was the one to say she wanted to go home because she was tired. There were so many simple things that I could do that made life easier. I was able to lift my leg to put my shoes and socks on rather than having to sit down and pull each leg over the opposite knee with my hand. I could run everywhere and I took full of advantage of this. (I literally ran everywhere for some time after getting off *The Biggest Loser*. Because I could! I kind of turned into Forrest Gump!) If I couldn't reach something I could jump to grab it or climb up on a chair without worrying about breaking it! One of the real standout things that I found myself being able to accomplish was to climb up on top of a roof. Just to know that I can do this makes me feel amazing. I will find any excuse to climb on to a roof – if someone has an antenna to fix, I'm your man!

Getting into the swing of these new activities and abilities actually took some time, though. It took the next six to 12 months for me to stop feeling hesitant about my actual weight: I would still put my hand down first when going to sit on a seat and apply pressure to make sure the seat could hold me before I sat on it properly; I would turn sideways to walk through turnstiles and doorways; and I would still go to oversized-clothing stores to look for clothing.

As I started to lose weight I realised that nothing is ever more important than working on yourself. Learning to put me first was one of the hardest changes I have ever had to make – hard because I wasn't used to it and it felt selfish. But somewhere along the journey I realised that it wasn't selfish at all, because I knew that being happy with the person I was would make me better for others and a better father.

Sometimes being selfish is the most selfless act you will ever do. By giving yourself the space to become deeply fulfilled and complete you pave a path of self-fulfilment for others to follow so they, too, can become beautiful and whole themselves.

On reflecting about the whole weight loss journey, I have never really come to terms with what bothered me more; the fact that I used to live my life at the level I did and never aim for more, or the fact that I was okay to live my life that way with never wanting more and just being okay with that.

The tragedy in life doesn't lie in not reaching your goal. The tragedy lies in having no goal to reach.
– Benjamin Mays

WORKSHOP: Putting yourself first

Putting you first is vital, especially for parents. If you think that
taking time out, away from your kids, to do a workout, visit
a gym or find a moment to relax, is selfish and impossible,
remember this: kids grow up and aspire to be like us, so if
we don't have control over our lives then our kids see this,
regardless of the lessons we give them. If we learn to love and
value ourselves, then the people around us will do the same.
It's one of the most amazing gifts you will ever be able to give.

Write down a list of things that you would like to do, to
take time out for yourself and recharge in order to see the
importance of you and 'you' time.

Shedding my skin suit *(Keep striving for your dreams)*

Stepping into post-Loser life reminded me of the dream I used to have as a child where I discovered I had a zip down the side of my body and my weight was merely a fat suit I could unzip and step out of. My *Biggest Loser* experience was kind of like my dream come true: I felt like I finally found that zipper and the slim me stepped out in what seemed a blink of an eye. The reality, though, was that I was trapped inside a skin suit.

After losing all the weight, I expected the fat suit to be replaced with a body that was tight, trim and packed with muscle. Boy, was I wrong! As the fat dropped away it left layers of excess skin. I still had boobs and an apron hanging over my belly. Psychologically this was devastating – and I did feel a little cheated that I'd lost weight but still had the flab; I still had the same bad body just a smaller version. This wasn't what I had dreamed about.

So I reseached and found a plastic and cosmetic surgeon to help me, Dr Mark Kohout. On our first appointment, we talked through the process of surgery and the possibilities of how I could fix my problem. Surgery of this kind is no minor operation – I was looking at several operations and hours of surgery to get the results I was after. It wasn't a decision to be taken lightly.

I began to research the procedure and reflect on what it would mean for me to have the excess skin removed. I realised that what I was hoping for was closure. I felt I needed the surgery because psychologically I was still the same obese person. I was proud of the fact that I had lost so much weight but I still had a body that looked exactly the same – the only difference was that I could fit into a medium shirt and size 34 pants instead of a 4XL shirt and size 52 pants.

After doing my research, thinking through things and getting opinions from four other surgeons, I really felt most comfortable with Dr Kohout. Together we began to plan the procedures. Two operations, five different procedures and 11 hours spent on an operating table over six weeks and my fat suit had been unzipped completely.

Dr Kohout did an amazing job, and although he knows he fixed my body I don't think he will ever know how he fixed my mind – my psychological state and body image. The surgery gave me the closure that I felt I earned and deserved as a part of losing all that weight. I may have scars, but I would much rather wear the scars of surgery than the scars of obesity I was otherwise left with.

It is very important if you are considering something like plastic surgery during or after your weight loss that you:

– Have finished losing all of your weight

– Are comfortable with the surgeon

– Are comfortable with the surgeon's past work, which you have checked out through photographs or by speaking with past clients.

To find an accredited plastic surgeon contact, Australian Society of Plastic Surgeons (*www.plasticsurgery.org.au*).

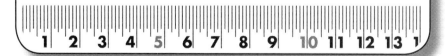

Unexpected changes *(Live your best life)*

When I said 'Let's change my world' that fateful day, I never realised how those words would strike home. As the saying goes, 'Be careful what you wish for, you just might get it'.

On 30 November 2006, my son Eden Harper (named after my Eden epiphany, and my saviour Bob Harper) was born. One of the greatest perks from losing weight that came with being a dad to two kids, was to be able to carry my two children around at the same time, without getting tired. And the best perk? Now when my kids say they want to be just like me, I can say I'm okay with that.

The freedom I have attained from a life of being weighed down, I know, spills over into my children. I know in my heart that they will grow to be free individuals, because I had the courage to change my life; to gain control of a life that I had never had any control over before.

Becoming a father again was just one of the many changes that took place in the year after becoming Australia's first-ever Biggest Loser. With the weight loss, came change: some positive, some negative. The positive changes were obvious – becoming more whole, happy and active as a father. I planned for and expected these positive changes, and they were amazing. It was the downside to losing weight and changing my life and lifestyle that I didn't expect. My relationships with my family and close friends were different; I also experienced resentment from people over my success.

WORKSHOP: Managing change

When you start to lose weight you may find that your relationships with people start to change. Friends may not understand why you don't want to go out for pizza and beer on Friday nights anymore, or conflict may arise in the household when family members or flatmates don't want to eat your 'diet' foods, and friends look at you as though you're being difficult when you're out for dinner and you put your special 'Can I have the dressing on the side?' order in.

Involve your family and friends in your weight loss by showing them how losing weight makes you a better partner, friend and person to them, get others involved in your new healthy way of living by suggesting you go for a walk or cycle with them or doing fun and active things as a way to socialise such as golf, throwing a Frisbee on the beach, a game of cricket at the park or joining a team sport such as indoor soccer. Think of some tactics that you can use to involve the people around you in your new lifestyle.

The biggest relationship that was impacted by my time on *The Biggest Loser* was my relationship with my wife, Sam.

When I went into the *Biggest Loser* house I felt Sam and I were on the same page – we were the best of mates, we were at the same place in life, we shared everything – yet when I returned we were both in different places. I had gone through a personal transformation. These personal changes, shifts in our perspectives and various events led to our separation three years later.

Quite often people who have been through relationship change, after or during weight loss, be it their own change or the change of partners, can blame the weight loss. This may not always be the cause; relationships can fail for lots of reasons. To help you prepare better for possible change within your relationships, take your partner, friends and family on the ride with you.

WORKSHOP: Strengthen your resolve

Always remain true to yourself and your goals. In your quest for a new you there might be a time when relationships shift or may become destructive or you may have trouble dealing with negativity from others. Keep yourself strong by reminding yourself of your goals and what you have achieved. Revisit the weight loss dreams and goals you wrote down in Part 1. Make a note of how far you have come and write down any new goals that you want to achieve.

Achievements so far

Congratulations, at the end of this section you have addressed your dreams and goals and started to look seriously at committing to your weight loss plans. With this part I hope you have:

✔ Written down positive thoughts about your life and had a go at tackling something you thought was too hard. Changing your mindset, changes the outcome.

✔ Listed what you want to achieve with your weight loss plans and looked deep into your heart to make these plans happen.

✔ Stripped down to your underwear and 'body mapped'.

✔ Listed the things you would like to do and put yourself first.

✔ Thought of some tactics to involve your family and friends in your weight loss goal.

✔ Revisited your weight loss dreams and goals and added new ones to your list.

THE NEW ~~ME~~ YOU

Where are you up to?

WEEK: **WEIGHT:**

Emotional state

Physical state

Challenges

Accomplishments

POSITIVE PLUS:

I feel great today because

I am amazing because

I will/am succeed/ing because

GOALS:

INSPIRATIONAL QUOTE:

PART 3

The New Me Program

Planning and preparing for The New You

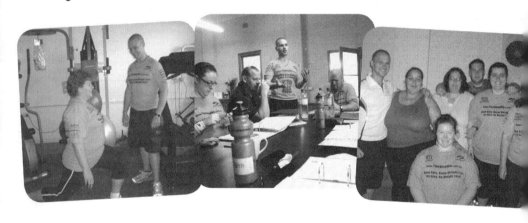

LEFT TO RIGHT: Me training with Sue Garret; Taking a New Me class with Fiona Dick, Geoff Tunks and Steve Ryan (our biggest male loser to date, 13.3 kg lost in 2 weeks); *The New Me*'s first ever group: me, Sharna and Margaret Bloom, Ben Orlanski, Sonia Dipardo, Anna Chiefello and Alida Dryer at the front. **OPPOSITE:** Me teaching the Move More component of *The New Me* program.

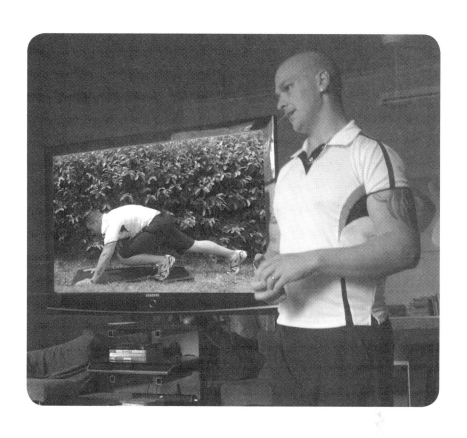

By failing to prepare,
you are preparing to fail.
— Benjamin Franklin

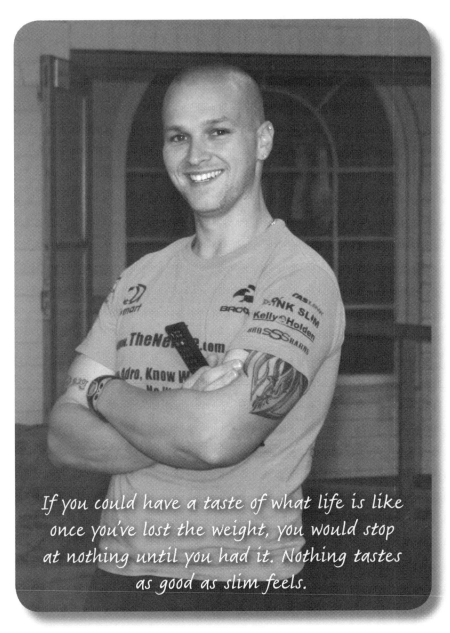

If you could have a taste of what life is like once you've lost the weight, you would stop at nothing until you had it. Nothing tastes as good as slim feels.

ABOVE: Proudly taking a class at *The New Me* (sitting at my lightest adult weight of about 81 kg).

Something I always tell people to do when I'm coaching them is to enjoy this weight loss journey because I'm going to do my best to make sure it's the last time you ever have to lose weight. You can lose weight fast and for good, and this part of the book is going to show you how.

After I won the title of Australia's first Biggest Loser I promised Australians that I was going to help them lose weight. And I have kept that promise. I am now a personal trainer, weight loss coach, motivational speaker and columnist for various magazines.

Wanting to lose weight, needing to lose weight, and then actually losing weight when you are clinically obese is not a simple task. Yes, it took a TV program to assist me to finally put my life on track, but I was able to make a true lifestyle change as a result. Since then, I have been inspired to create my own weight loss retreat in the tradition of classic health and fitness spas that date back to Roman times. 'The New Me Weight Loss Retreat' on Victoria's beautiful Mornington peninsula, is a revitalising, special place where people are given an opportunity to make a profound change in their lives with the help of my program, emotional support and weight loss know-how based on the lessons (and pitfalls) of my own weight loss story. It took 18 months to get things ready and opened on 16 March 2008. It's an education facility, teaching practical lifestyle modification techniques to help people move over to a healthier lifestyle (and assist with weight loss). It is also a retreat that aims to inspire people to become all they have ever wanted to be, find themselves and begin to choose life.

REAL LIFE TRANSFORMATIONS WITH THE NEW ME PROGRAM

Caroline Garrick, 38

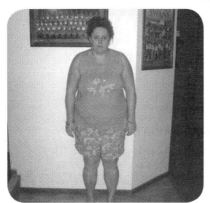 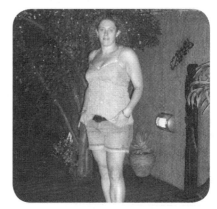

Total weight lost on The New Me Program

43 kilograms (13 kilograms lost in four weeks at The New Me Weight Loss Retreat; 30 kilograms continuing with the program at home, afterwards)

The old me (123 kilograms)

Before going to The New Me Weight Loss Retreat, I was at an all-time low; feeling depressed and unhappy with the way I looked and felt about myself. None of my clothes fitted me and I felt embarrassed for my kids to have a mum who was so overweight and felt I was not setting a good example. I started thinking about some form of surgery before finding The New Me Program.

The New Me (80 kilograms and a goal of losing another 5 kilograms to reach my ideal weight)

I feel and look healthy. I have so much energy and love that I can shop for clothes that fit me at the stores I would never have been able to shop at before.

Biggest weight loss lesson

Prior to The New Me I had an all-or-nothing mentality. Now, if I have a bad day I don't let it go further than that and am straight back on track the next day.

Mac Sarnelli, 34

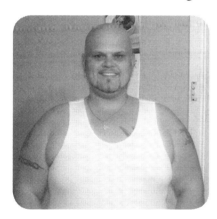 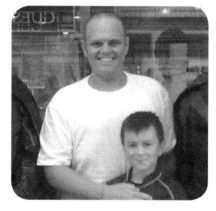

Total weight lost on The New Me Program

93 kilograms (13 kilograms at The New Me Weight Loss Retreat; 30 kilograms continuing with the program at home afterwards; the rest beforehand with Adro's eating and exercise advice)

The old me (206 kilograms)

The old me was a very angry negative person, who always believed that you take everything for its worst and then it can only get better.

And I thought it worked. It helped with the loneliness that only food and no exercise can comfort. My weight affected my life in every way: I had no energy to enjoy a game with the kids, it was only for a half-hour and then I needed the rest of the weekend to recover; no sex drive; no clothes to show the real me; the list went on . . .

Initially I had the attitude of just starve or eat carrots and it will be okay. Like my brother, I thought there must be a genetic reason that stopped me from successfully losing weight. Once I ran out of excuses for not going to my brother's retreat, I decided to give it a go with an open mind and take on board anything that they had to teach me. What I was doing wasn't working and the trainers in my local gym told me to follow their regime and it would be okay . . . but it wasn't. At the retreat, it was a counsellor who made it all click and with the help and support of my brother and assistance from the trainers, my life has started to turn around.

What keeps me going is being able to go into one of my favourite clothing stores and now being able to buy something off the rack.

The New Me (108 kilograms and still falling)
Happy to be alive and reversing my fate from an early obesity-related death. I am happier than I have been in a long time and can now go on 'throw-up' rides and not have to worry about not fitting in the chair. It is exciting now to be able to run; it makes a good start to the morning (well most mornings). I can't wait to go running with my sisters after they have come back from The New Me Weight Loss Retreat. Sometimes it does pay to have a brother!

Biggest weight loss lesson
There are no excuses, just choices.

Matt Quinten, 34

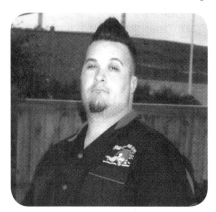 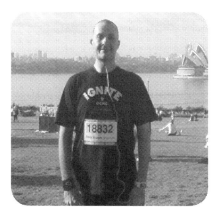

Total weight lost on The New Me Program
78 kilograms (in twelve months)

The old me (165 kilograms)

When I first met Adro we were both big fellas; both medically categorised as morbidly obese. I had been this way my entire adult life. Our friendship formed through cars. On weekends, a fast-food restaurant car park was a convenient meeting place for all the car enthusiasts, where we would meet and eat before cruising onto the next junk-food joint. During the week, being busy, convenient foods were the order of the day.

I reached in excess of 170 kilograms, by making uninformed food choices, choosing fast food and not exercising. Standing in front of a mirror without a shirt on, moved me to tears.

Seeing Adro win *The Biggest Loser* inspired me by demonstrating that transformation can happen. I wanted to become my own New Me. With a combination of lap band surgery and Adro's exercise and eating advice I lost almost half my body weight in 12 months.

The New Me (87 kilograms)

I can proudly say I am no longer overweight and enjoy being fit. I have motivation to incorporate exercise into my life. I feel better physically and think more clearly. I set, and achieved, my goal to run in the City to Surf, a 14-kilometre fun run in Sydney. And have since completed other fun runs. I now train up to six days a week, sometimes twice a day. My resting heart rate has shifted from 95 to 42 beats per minute. I have lowered my blood pressure and blood sugar levels.

Biggest weight loss lesson

For me, it all started with the acceptance of the position I was in. I started slowly, taking a little step at a time, and the results snowballed. Acceptance leads to motivation, motivation leads to action, and action leads to results.

One of the key things I realised and now teach at 'The New Me' is the need to identify that your old ways aren't working; the old system didn't work. The key is creating a new system and then making that your life – leaving as many things as possible from the old system out of the new system.

You need to do the opposite of what caused you to gain weight in order to lose weight.

It's this premise that inspired the creation of the system I use in my life, as a weight loss coach, and at The New Me Weight Loss Retreat. I have developed a program focusing on what I found to be the three major elements to weight loss: food intake, exercise and attitude. My program is based on three key principles: Eat Smart, Move More, Think Thin. These three things helped me lose weight and are the principles I live by to keep the weight off for good. Now it's time for you to discover 'The New You'.

Getting started

*You can lose weight fast
and for good.*

There are four important things to remember to get you in the right headspace for your New Me journey. Be ready to . . .

✔ GET started – Once and for all, this is it, get ready to get started on the program.

✔ GET fit – This involves being aware of not only your physical fitness but also your mental and emotional fitness.

✔ GET real – It took you a lot of time and effort to gain weight (maybe not consciously). So be realistic about the time and effort you will need to put in to lose the weight.

✔ GET focused– Believe in yourself and the work that you are doing will bring results.

Before you begin, there are a few formalities that need to be taken care of.

- ## See your doctor

Before starting any exercise program, please consult with your doctor and let them know what you are intending to do. Make sure you get a medical all clear to begin.

- ## Photograph yourself

You may not like this, but I would encourage you to take some photos of yourself. This is important to give you a memory of how far you've come and as a tool to look at your progress to motivate you if you feel like giving up. Plus once you lose weight you will wish that you had the before photos to show everyone and yourself where you came from.

Take the photos yourself or get your partner or a friend to take them. Take two types of shots: one fully clothed and one wearing only your underwear. For the clothed shot, wear just one layer. Take photos, front, side and rear on. You want to see the changes to your body as you lose weight from all angles, not everyone loses weight from the same spots. Put in the date by holding up the front page of the day's newspaper or simply a piece of paper with the date written on it, to have a record of the day you decided to change.

- ## Weigh in

If, like me, you stopped weighing yourself after it reached a certain point, because you didn't want to have to face the climbing number anymore, I think it's important to face the truth. Remember, you're doing this because it doesn't matter so much where you are, it matters where you are going – and that is down on the scales.

It's important to have one set day for a controlled weigh-in. You need to control the weigh-in by removing any variables and making the weigh-in as consistent as possible. For example, every Monday morning, with no clothes on as soon as you wake up and after you have been to the toilet. It's best to stick to one weigh-in each week, under the same circumstances, to give you the best idea of what's really happening with your weight.

- ## Try on

If stepping on the scales is just too much for you at this point, take some notes on how you feel and look in a particular outfit and use this as your measure of progress – meaning each week instead of having a weigh-in, you have a 'try-on' where you try this same outfit on and note if it feels looser and where it feels different.

- ## Measure up

A simple measure of your weight loss and a quick indicator of your health (because stomach fat is a risk factor for disease) is a measurement of your waist. You can do this in two ways:

1. Use a belt and note which hole fits you each week. If you can't find a belt that fits, simply get yourself an old belt and make holes in it further along – you will reach those holes that are already there, soon!

2. Use a measuring tape, the kind you use for sewing, and take your waist measurement by wrapping the tape halfway between your lowest rib and the top of your hipbone, roughly in line with your belly button. Don't breathe in or suck your stomach in; breathe normally and measure on the out breath. And make sure the tape is snug but not tight.

Once you've taken your photos, you can stick them in your Transformation Journal (see Part 4: The New Me Tool Kit), as well as recording all of the measurements. Grab your pen and diary and mark your weekly appointment to weigh in or try on, and measure up. And next to your weekly appointment, to set you off on the right foot, write, 'Goodbye old me, New Me here I come!'

WORKSHOP: Measure up

Storing excess weight around your midsection means you're likely to have fat deposits surrounding your internal organs, which is not good for your health, and increases your risk of developing a lifestyle-related chronic disease, such as heart disease, some cancers and Type 2 diabetes. For most Australians a waist measurement of over 94 centimetres for men and 80 centimetres for women means you are at increased risk of developing a chronic disease. If your waist measurement is over 102 centimetres for men and 88 centimetres for women, your risk greatly increases. For more information, and a free printable tape measure, you can visit *www.measureup.gov.au*

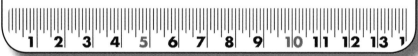

One way to get thin is to re-establish a purpose in life. – Cyril Connolly

We need to focus on ourselves in order to lose the weight and regain our health and life, however, once we feel full again by sharing our success with others we commit to a purpose larger than ourselves. This shift allows us to change our focus. Now I feed my spirit instead of my stomach and maintaining a healthy and active lifestyle is a simple and easy act of self-love.

Let's get started.

Turn your dreams into goals

You need to take a moment to think of where you're going. Now everyone dreams, right? Before you think, 'Goal setting, been there done that, boring!', think of a goal as a short-term dream.

Let's take a moment to dream.

WORKSHOP: Starting your new life

List the differences in life, and as a person, that you are hoping to notice between your current life and the new life you're starting today.

Goals are dreams with deadlines.
— Diana Scharf Hunt

1 2 3 4 5 6 7 8 9 10 11 12 13

Setting small, realistic goals is the key to successful goal setting – let's call them Mini Goals. Setting Mini Goals instead of saying 'I have to lose 60 kilograms (132 pounds)' is a lot more achievable. It is a lot less daunting to lose 1 kilogram (2.2 pounds) at a time, 60 times over. It becomes manageable both in your head and on your body.

Have you ever heard the saying, 'How do you eat an elephant? … A little bit at a time.'? This is how you need to approach your weight loss: one step at a time. Just trust that as long as you keep taking a step forwards you will get to the top.

> Thinking of how far you have to go is overwhelming. Focusing on what you can do right now to help with your weight loss is empowering.

Don't stop goal setting after your pen leaves the paper on the worksheet or in your journal. Goal setting is something you need to do throughout your whole day, every day and your entire life. Goals and dreams inspire us and give us something positive to focus on. So dream big!

> Aim for the moon, so if you fall short you still reach the stars.
> – W Clements

WORKSHOP: Set your goals

What is your current weight?   kg/pounds

What is your goal weight?   kg/pounds

How much weight is this to lose?   kg/pounds

What is your time frame to lose the weight?   weeks

How many kilograms per week is this?   kg/pounds

My Mini Goal is to lose   kg/pounds per week!

What is something physical you would like to be able to do in?

4 weeks:

12 months:

5 years:

1 2 3 4 5 6 7 8 9 10 11 12 13 1

Committing to your goals

Committing to doing everything possible to reach your dream goal is a crucial step. To do this we need to commit to doing the opposite of what causes us to be overweight. You must make a full-fledged commitment to not let anything stand in between the old and The New You, and pledge that failure isn't an option.

To help with your commitment you're about to sign a contract. The purpose of this contract is so that you take the agreement to reach your goal weight seriously; to make a conscious decision that you are about to change your habits, lifestyle and fitness, and, as a welcomed effect of this, you will reduce your weight; and to make yourself accountable by making a promise to yourself.

This is a contract that will last forever and the only way to breach it is to give up on yourself.

The fact that you have also committed your goals to paper will give you more chance of achieving them. Studies have shown that those who commit their goals to paper are the most successful. One major study found that only three per cent of people are likely to achieve their goals, and the only difference between the people who do achieve their goals and the ones who don't is that the successful ones write their goals down.

Take the contract seriously, because we want it to be the last time you ever have to make such a pledge. Date the contract and then once it is completed, cut it out or make a copy and put it somewhere where you will see it every day. Read it at least once a day, each morning. This is a great way to reaffirm your goals and commitment.

Getting a partner, friend or family member to witness it is to show another person how serious you are and to gain their support. Sharing your commitment is important because we seem to find it easy to back out of a commitment we have made only to ourselves but think twice before backing out on a commitment we have made to another person. And gaining support from another person is important because there may be times when you want to let yourself down, and that special someone hopefully won't let you.

Take a photocopy of the following pages with the blank contract and use it to write up your own contract.

Dedication or inspiration is the ease in which you reach success when your goals and values align, and motivation is the force necessary to reach success when they don't.
— as taught by Dr John Demartini

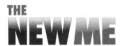

NEW ME

Personal Agreement Contract

This contract is set into place on the _____ day of _____

in _____ .

I, _____ , have created this agreement and promised on this day to make a commitment to adjusting my current lifestyle in ways that are beneficial to my health, wellness and weight.

I promise myself that I will do everything in my power to reach my goal weight of _____ kilograms/pounds, which from this point will mean achieving my Mini Goal of _____ kilograms/pounds per week.

I will enjoy my commitment to better health and fitness and I will seek a diet and activity plan that I am in control of so that it will lessen my chances of not being happy with what someone has created for me. This will enable me to make this my strongest and final effort at gaining control of my weight and reaching my goal weight by _____ / _____ / _____ . I know that this is a realistic goal and so long as I keep at it I will achieve this in the set time.

I will find activities and exercises that I enjoy so that I can make this time of my life fun and memorable, and so I will want to continue each day.

I will seek help from, but not rely on, my family and friends to get me through this, knowing now that I have the power and ability to make my own dreams come true.

I will learn to be motivated and make better food choices to enable me to overcome cravings; and I will keep a food diary to help me identify and battle areas of the week where I struggle with my diet choices.

I will measure my progress regularly and reward myself for each Mini Goal I achieve; but these rewards will not be food!

I am committing now, to myself, that if I struggle or stray from my better diet choices I WILL NOT GIVE UP! I will learn that these temptations are a part of life that I will be dealing with forever, so the sooner I learn to accept and adapt to them the better I will respond to these situations.

And, finally, I will make the correct adjustments to my past and present so that this change becomes a lifestyle change that I enjoy and will continue throughout my life.

I will do everything in my power to Eat Smart, Move More and Think Thin.

I will reach my goal this time because:

_____

_____

_____

_____

_____

_____

_____

Signature _____

Date _____

My support (name printed) _____

Signature _____

Date _____

I would like to congratulate you on making the commitment to yourself and to your dreams and goals. Now it's time for a bit of self-reflection.

Why weight?

Once we know the why we begin to find the how.

The next step towards creating The New You is to ask why you are overweight and why you want to lose weight. I truly believe that the make-up of successful weight loss and keeping the weight off is a 100 per cent effort made up as a combination of:

- **50 per cent within you (psychologically, emotionally);**
- **30 per cent diet (the foods we eat and what we know about them); and**
- **20 per cent exercise and activity.**

This is why you need to spend as much time looking within, as you do looking outside at diet and exercise. You need to discover that something inside that makes you 'click', that finally makes you go, 'I finally get why I am overweight and what I have to do to change it.' (Things clicked for me when I realised I'd been fooling myself by thinking I had a time problem, not a weight problem; it clicked that I was overweight because of issues I was holding onto not because of a lack of time to exercise and eat right, which I used as an excuse.)

This may be hard to digest, but you have to acknowledge that you worked hard to

*get to the weight you are today. You didn't
just wake up overweight one day.*

Once you have acknowledged this, you can get to work putting in the same amount of effort to reverse the process; to switch from unconsciously gaining weight to consciously losing weight. Because although you don't consciously want to be the weight you are, on some unconscious level you do; you're receiving some pay-off from it – whether that's having an excuse to fall back on for areas of your life that aren't working or not being in a relationship or being afraid to step out of your comfort zone.

You need to own the problem in order to own the solution. Once you have owned the solution you can truly own success. And you will love this feeling of self-power.

WORKSHOP: Identify the real causes

Put time and thought into answering the following questions. You're the only person who needs to see these so be completely honest. If you're not honest with yourself then the only person who will suffer is you.

How did I become overweight?

_____

Why am I struggling with my weight?

_____

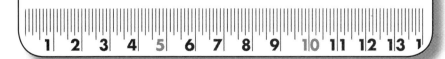

By bringing the reasons you struggle with your weight to the light it helps you to fight them. You can't fight what you can't see now, can you?

Once you have identified some reasons for why you struggle to lose weight, you can get on with removing the influences that sabotage your weight loss. One of the most influential things that will determine your success is recognising and dealing with sabotage – from yourself and from others.

An example of self-sabotage is being afraid of success so you binge eat every time you get close to achieving a goal. An example of sabotage from others, which may or may not be intentional, is continuing to bring junk food into the house when you've committed to giving up junk food. I really believe love can be a big sabotage – from parents who love us with food to friends and family feeling insecure if we were to change.

Reducing, replacing or removing the sabotaging influences in your life requires self-discipline from the start. But it is necessary to give yourself your best chance at losing weight.

Remember that this is all about you being the one who can do this, and you gaining the knowledge to empower yourself with the tools for success.

Dealing with our sources of sabotage needn't be as dramatic as it sounds. Quite often, it's just about raising our awareness and changing our habits. It's the bad or non-beneficial habits that we need to identify and replace with good, more beneficial ones. You will find it easier to think that you are swapping habits rather than getting rid of them.

Identifying the problems
in some cases is more work
than solving them.

WORKSHOP: Swap sabotages for solutions

List your sabotages and possible solutions or strategies to deal with each one:

Sabotages:

_____

_____

Solutions:

_____

_____

1 2 3 4 5 6 7 8 9 10 11 12 13 1

With all of those sabotaging forces out of the way, let's look at why you want to lose weight.

- Being overweight or obese puts you at an increased risk of: heart disease, stroke, high blood pressure, insulin resistance, pre-diabetes, Type 2 diabetes, some cancers, sleep apnoea, gall bladder disease, osteoarthritis and polycystic ovarian syndrome (PCOS).
- Being fit and a healthy weight is your best protection against disease and your best shot at living longer.

So why do you want to lose weight? The obvious answer is because you want to look and feel better, but you need to probe a little deeper. Why? Because it's the internal motivating factors that work best to keep you on track. For example, take an external motivation, such as losing weight to fit into an outfit for an upcoming party or a bride losing weight for her wedding day. Once the external event you were losing weight for arrives and ends what is going to drive you to keep going? An internal reason stays with you irrespective of what happens externally. One example of an internal motivator is wanting to be the best parent you can be to your children.

If you're not going to do this for yourself, then do it for someone you love; you will find it harder to let that person down, than you would yourself.

Another example of a lasting motivation is your health. Try to focus more on the health aspect of the lifestyle change rather than just the weight you wish to lose. Get excited at the prospect of what your new life will hold.

WORKSHOP: Changing your life

Think of how losing weight will change different areas of your life. The possibilities of a healthier, happier and thinner life are exciting and endless.

Why do I want to lose weight and be healthy?

_____

_____

How will losing weight change my life?

_____

_____

Who will The New Me be?

_____

_____

| 1 | 2 | 3 | 4 | 5 | 6 | 7 | 8 | 9 | 10 | 11 | 12 | 13 | 1 |

Okay, that's enough self-reflection for now. Let's get down to the nitty-gritty of how to lose weight. Time to Eat Smart, Move More and Think Thin.

EAT SMART

Learning how to **eat smart** will empower you with the necessary knowledge about the best foods and eating habits for a healthy weight and a healthy life.

Learning to eat smart is a process; if we knew how to eat smart, we wouldn't have a problem with our weight. So you need to draw on what you have already learnt from the (I'm guessing many) previous diets you've tried, toss out the things that don't work for you and build up your knowledge about the things that will work for you. The first step in this learning process is to create a smart diet.

STEP 1 – To eat smart you need to diet smart

Diet has become a bit of a dirty word, but a diet is necessary to begin; it gives you training wheels while you're learning to eat on your own, by giving you a set of guidelines to work with.

But keep in mind that *the goal is not to rely on a diet* because that wouldn't be smart as you wouldn't be able to sustain the diet (it is only human to get bored of a restricted or stringent diet regime). Some people also lose the weight (or some of the weight) they'd set out to lose and then revert back to their old way of eating.

Going on a diet implies that we can get off it. And you can't. A diet only gives us two options: on or off, whereas you can't get 'off' a better way of eating because it's the way you are. Successful and permanent weight loss means swapping the bad habits for good.

Going on a diet is a lot like going on a holiday: you're stressed out and you need a break, you get time off work, break free and live this different and relaxed way of life, and de-stress. But, upon your return everything slips right back into the old ways and you've learnt nothing because you've gone back to being stressed out. The same is true for weight loss: you need to lose weight, you go on a diet, lose weight, then return back to your old ways of eating and go back to the weight you were, or more! In order to not end up regaining weight you need to change things about the way you eat and live before returning back to your normal life.

Remember, the objective is to think of a diet as a tool to get you started while you are learning about the best foods to eat. Then, you can modify the diet to make it a way of eating that you can stick to for life.

A kick start

TIP   First, you make smart diet choices that complement weight loss; then you make smart food choices to complement a healthy lifestyle and weight maintenance.

STEP 2 – To eat smart you need to get smart about what food is really for

The next step in the learning process is to remind ourselves about the function of food. Food and drink are our fuel – to give us energy for activity, to assist bodily functions and feed our brains. Many of us struggle with our weight because we eat for so many reasons other than to simply fuel up. We need to change our emotional connection to food. We need to fall out of love with food!

WORKSHOP: Food reasons

Be honest with yourself and jot down some of the things that you think food is for? Don't think of your answers as silly, right or wrong. This is the time to nip some of your old ways of thinking in the bud, and regardless of how silly you think your answers may be, it's better to have a silly answer solved than a smart answer not solved. I have jotted a few things down to get you started, simply circle the relevant ones and add to the list.

To make me happy

So I have something to do when I go out

Something to talk over

Something to have wine with

To have with movies or while watching TV

To help when I'm upset

Something to keep me awake when I'm driving

_____

_____

_____

| 1 | 2 | 3 | 4 | 5 | 6 | 7 | 8 | 9 | 10 | 11 | 12 | 13 | 1 |

Now that you have learnt, or reminded yourself, that food is fuel and nothing else, you need to look at your food choices.

The rest of the world lives to eat,
while I eat to live. – Socrates

STEP 3 – To eat smart you need to make smart food choices

The smartest food choices are the ones that are smartest for your weight loss and your lifestyle. You will learn all about the smartest foods for weight loss in the Eat Smart Diet in Part 4: The New Me Tool Kit, but I bet you already know what foods are not smart for you; those trigger foods that you tell yourself you just can't resist and can't stop eating!

WORKSHOP: Trigger foods

Make a list of your trigger foods. You know the ones, the must-have foods that you just can't imagine living without, the ones you just have to have as soon as you see or think about them! (Mmmm, your mouth is watering already):

1 2 3 4 5 6 7 8 9 10 11 12 13 1

Now that you have a list of your typical not-so-smart/trigger foods, the next step is setting up a space where you have the most chance of success.

STEP 4 – To eat smart you need to create a smart food environment

One of the easiest ways of making sure that you only have good food around to choose from is to, well, only have good food around to choose from! I know that sounds straightforward and simple, but it's true. The reason to do this is to save yourself from those moments of weakness when you crave those trigger foods – you'll either have to go out and get them or go without – meaning you can't accidentally eat crap; by choosing to go out and actually get it makes it a conscious decision to actually eat it, eradicating the, 'Oops, I ate it because it was there' excuse, or the, 'Did I just eat that whole packet of biscuits?' realisation after you've mindlessly snacked while watching a movie.

> **TIP** Getting rid of all the bad foods from your pantry and fridge will stop you from 'accidentally' grabbing a chocolate biscuit when you get up during the 8.30 movie to make yourself a cuppa.

So, get to it! Go to your cupboards, fridge and freezer, and get rid of your not-so-smart/trigger foods. Make sure you don't leave any foods from your trigger food list.

Practise the same habit with leftovers. While it's great to keep leftover food to save money and time, if you're going to go back and keep picking at it instead of putting it away for tomorrow's meal, leftover food is better off in the bin, or the freezer if you must keep it. It's common for mothers to comment on how they end up finishing off their children's meals and most of us have been conditioned to not waste food.

> **TIP** It's not bad to throw extras away. Would you rather it go to waste, or go to your waist?

If you cannot totally commit to removing all temptation from the house – you may feel it's too extreme or not want to take away treats from the rest of the family (keep in mind that it is better for their health, too) or feel you need biscuits in the cupboard for when guests come over (keep in mind, you can just as easily give them healthy treats with their cuppa or drink) – straightaway that is fine. (Although be honest with yourself over the reason for this – are they excuses or genuine reasons? You decide.) Perhaps start off with removing just one trigger food or substituting your trigger foods for healthier versions that contain fewer calories.

Remember, a little effort is better than no effort at all. But the harder you go, the faster you will get results and the less time it will take you to reach your goal.

This brings us to the last step in eating smart, and that is learning the art of substitution.

STEP 5 – To eat smart you need to make smart substitutions

I'm sure you'd agree it's better to consume more of the good foods rather than less of the bad foods?

The Eat Smart principle is all about finding smart ways to eat within your everyday environment while still losing weight and still being able to enjoy good food without overdosing on calories. Once you fine-tune your food adaptation skills, you will be armed with the invaluable knowledge of the smartest way to make up your meals – a skill that you will use for the rest of your life – from substituting single ingredients to lower the calories or fat content of recipes, to knowing what to substitute when ordering at a restaurant, to switching to a smarter product choice when doing the groceries.

A simple example of substitution is something that you have probably already started doing. That is replacing full-fat products with low-fat products; or substituting normal foods with diet foods.

A word on diet foods

While diet versions of favourite foods that are high in fat, sugar and calories can be a great way to reduce calorie intake, there are a couple of things about diet foods that I'd like to point out, so you can make an informed choice about the best foods to eat:

- Nothing is better or more nutritious than fresh whole food that is closest to its natural form (for example, a packet of apple-filled biscuits looks nothing like an apple, therefore is nothing like its natural form). As diet guru Dr John Tickell says, minimise HI (human intervention).

- Diet foods may contain preservatives and additives. Whether you choose to consume these is a personal preference. You can find out more about the possible side effects of additives and preservatives from a health practitioner.

- Diet foods that are remakes of normal 'bad' foods should be avoided while losing weight; use them to prevent weight gain once you have reached your goal or are close to it.

- Fat-free may not mean low calories or sugar-free so read the ingredients list carefully. When you are choosing low-fat items be sure you're not getting a huge sugar content in the product as a substitute for the fat.

- Just because something is low in calories, doesn't mean it is low in salt (sodium) and sugar – sugar can go under many names which you may miss, such as brown sugar, corn sweetener, corn syrup, dextrose, fructose, fruit juice concentrates, glucose, high-fructose corn syrup, honey, inverted sugar, lactose, maltose, malt, syrup, molasses, raw sugar, sucrose, sugar syrup.

- Diet foods can lull you into a false sense of security – 'It's diet food so I can eat as much as I like'. Whether you eat healthy food, diet food or bad food – eat too much of it and you will gain weight. Eating diet food does not mean you can eat more; it means you're better off at the end of the day than if you eat the same amount of non-diet food.

- Just because something says 'health bar' doesn't mean it is better for you – it may still have the same, if not more, calories and/or fat content.

continued

- There is no such thing as diet chocolate. (Food for thought: exercise releases the same endorphins as chocolate.)
- Oven-roasted nuts are not roasted; they are deep-fried in an oven.
- 'Lite' could simply mean light in colour, weight, texture or anything else other than light in fat or calories.

When you are trying to lose weight it is important to realise that you need to break the habits that contributed to your original weight gain. If chocolate, for example, was your weakness, then you would still be succumbing to that temptation, regardless of the fact that you are eating a diet version and therefore not breaking your habit.

Here are some examples of food substitution ideas. Using your calorie-counting book (see Part 4: The New Me Tool Kit), fill in at least four more, then create a bigger list in your weight loss journal or on a chart you can copy and hang in your kitchen. Be sure to include some substitutions for your favourite treats. You can refer back to this table in the future when you need a quick guide on how to save calories. Once you refer to it enough, these food swaps will become second nature.

Smart Substitutions

Original item/calories	Substitute item/calories	Calories saved
1 glass cordial/85	1 glass diet cordial/4	81
Vegetable oil (1 tbsp)/159	Oil spray (2–3 second spray)/33	126
Oil spray (2–3 seconds)/33	Low-cal spray (2–3 second spray)/2.5	30.5
200 grams full-fat yoghurt/180	200 grams fat-free yoghurt/94	86
1 tsp butter/36	1 tsp light olive oil spread/25	11
1 full-strength beer/135	1 low-carb beer/107 1 no carb beer/88	28
Large whole egg/95	Egg white of large egg/16	79
1 serving jelly/86	1 serving diet jelly/5	81
Coke (600 ml)/258	Coke Zero(600 ml)/2	256

TIP Modify your favourite recipes. Another example of substitution is switching ingredients in recipes to lower the overall fat and calorie content – this is what the Eat Smart Recipes (see Part 4) are all about. Why not start practising by creating your own Eat Smart Recipes?

WORKSHOP: Tips to help you eat smart

- **Fall out of love with food:** Learn to enjoy food instead of having a love affair with food! Food is for filling up the fuel tank not for satisfying feelings and emotions. Your body doesn't desire or receive pleasure from the treats you eat. It's your mind that's receiving pleasure. (I bet your car doesn't get excited when you're pulling into a petrol station hoping it's going to get premium petrol!) Your desperate desires for indulgent foods are self-created; the flavours you associate with desire are learnt. Food is simply fuel for the most amazing machine on Earth: your body. So fill it up with foods that take care of it, not foods that satisfy your self-created desires.

- **Eat slowly:** Slow down when eating as it takes around 20 minutes for your brain to register that you are full. Try putting your cutlery down after you take each bite, eating with your opposite hand to slow you down or eating with chopsticks or small cutlery like teaspoons or dessert forks.

- **Practise the God-versus-guilt theory:** If the urge to have a treat is too great, take one tablespoon of the treat (or a bite or mini portion), leave it until the end of the meal to trick your brain into thinking that it has been satisfied by that particular food, and then eat that one spoonful savouring every sensation in your mouth as you eat it, remembering that the first bite is GODLY and the rest will make you feel GUILTY.

- **Eat small meals often:** Eating small meals and often keeps your metabolism burning and helps prevent you from gorging when you do get around to eating because you're so hungry – you know that feeling where you can't get enough in fast enough! Avoid eating one to two large meals later in the day, thinking that if you eat less in the day it won't matter what you eat at night. Sumo wrestlers who train all day and only eat once a day for no more than half an hour do this to slow their metabolism down in order to gain weight. To eat less, eat off a bread plate or leave some food behind.

- **Organise everything:** You don't want to be caught off guard when temptation hits. If you prepare snacks for the day you won't be tempted to get junk food or stop at drive-throughs.

- **Drink water:** You cannot underestimate the value of drinking a lot of water. Studies have shown that 80 per cent of the time we are feeling hungry we are actually thirsty. Learn the value of developing a drinking habit (of water, of course!) and drink water before and during your meals to help fill you up.

- **Brush your teeth after eating:** Don't rinse the tooth-paste out properly so it makes food after brushing taste bad.

- **Stop picking:** Try chewing gum or snacking on celery (it takes more calories to digest celery than the amount of calories contained in the celery) when preparing meals and children's school lunches. This will stop you from picking at the crust you cut off or whatever it is that you may otherwise pop into your mouth.

- **Prepare for the event of emotional eating:** Having strategies in place such as the use of affirmations, a buddy or someone you can call when you need to talk, taking a bath, lighting a candle and reading an inspirational book or writing in a journal, or having a favourite funny movie on hand helps you to choose a constructive strategy instead of food while you're *continued* emotionally vulnerable. By planning a handful of self-nurturing ways that you can use to deal with depression, stress, frustration, low self-esteem, sadness, rejection and so on, you can help yourself feel better without eating food. This will equip you to respond rather than react, and build up your skills of taking care of yourself in non-food ways.

- **Always question yourself:** Are you going to the fridge because you are hungry or bored? Are you eating when you're actually thirsty (dehydrated)? Are you opening your wallet to get money for junk food?

- **Change your food focus:** Stop making food the focus of events and start to focus more on the fun things that you have special occasions for such as making a special day for the birthday person or spending time with family at a family function. Plan active get-togethers like bowling, barefoot bowling, picnics and a sporting game in the park, putt-putt golf, bush walking and so on.

- **Never reward yourself with food:** Never never, ever ever — with the emphasis on 'Never'. Reaching your goal weight is your reward.

Add some more of your own tips for eating smart. These may be tips you've read or heard or things that have worked for you before.

1 2 3 4 5 6 7 8 9 10 11 12 13 1

Achievements so far

Congratulations, at the end of this section you have now been completely honest with yourself about your motives and reasons for weight loss plus you will have learnt how to 'Eat Smart'. With this part I hope you have:

✔ Listed the differences in life, and as a person, that you are hoping to notice between your current life and the new life you plan to start.

✔ Set your goals to get started on The New Me Program.

✔ Written and signed your own personal agreement contract. You have formally committed to your weight loss plan.

✔ Been completely honest about your weight issues and bravely moved towards owning your problems in order to own the solution to them.

✔ Learnt how to swap sabotage for solutions and come up with strategies to counteract difficult influences in your life.

✔ Thought about how losing weight will change different areas of your life – for good.

✔ Been honest with yourself about what you use food for.

✔ Made a list of your trigger foods.

✔ Worked out smart foods to substitute with the not-so-smart foods.

✔ Created your own 'Eat Smart' tips to help target your weight loss goals.

THE NEW ME YOU

Where are you up to?

WEEK: **WEIGHT:**

Emotional state

Physical state

Challenges

Accomplishments

POSITIVE PLUS:

I feel great today because

I am amazing because

I will/am succeed/ing because

GOALS:

INSPIRATIONAL QUOTE:

MOVE MORE

Simply **move more** to burn more. Of course, this isn't a revolutionary idea; it's pretty straightforward. But if you remember to up your activity level each day and keep reminding yourself that this activity is necessary to help burn up calories then questions of walking to the corner shop rather than driving or taking the stairs rather than the lift will be easily answered. Keep repeating the simple mantra 'move more to burn more, burn more to lose more', to inspire yourself to take the active path every day.

Rethink the way you approach exercise and movement. The higher the heart rate and the longer it stays there, the more calories you burn. How easy is that? Simply move more to keep upping your heart rate. Move it to lose it.

> *TIP* Wearing a heart rate monitor during your day can be a good move motivator, by way of seeing that the more you increase your heart rate, by being more active and exercising, the more calories you burn.

*Swap a sedentary life
for an active life.*

Fast weight loss is possible if you put in the effort

The conventional idea for weight loss is working out three times a week and following a sensible diet plan to obtain a loss of ½ to 1 kilogram (1.1 to 2.2 pounds) per week, however I believe this restricts you with limits. If we're told that it is only possible to achieve a set result and if we hear it enough we set our capabilities around this expectation. My theory, and one I put into practice is: why get these results for this much effort when if you do twice the work you will get twice the result? As long as you remain healthy in the process you can push beyond the limits that are being set by the mainstream.

I told myself that if I worked out six times a week, I should lose 1–2 kilograms (2.2–4.4 pounds) per week, and if I was to work out nine times a week I should lose 2–3 kilograms (4.4–6.6 pounds) per week, and if I worked out 12 times I would lose 3–4 kilograms (6.6–8.8 pounds) per week. And so on. This is how I lost my weight so quickly and what I base The New Me training program on. Go twice as hard for half the time, rather than half as hard for twice the time.

Please note: When undertaking a new exercise routine or even increasing the intensity of your normal routine, it is very important that you **find a balance that is practical and safe for you**. Exercising at the intensity and frequency I did may not be right for you. Always consult with your doctor before undertaking any new exercise program to be sure it is right for your situation and your particular health position.

The first major step is to stop living the lazy life by moving more each day.

STEP 1 – To move more you need to move more

Sounds simple but it's something we seem to have lost sight of. This doesn't mean go to the gym more, it means get up off your butt and get involved with everyday things that require you to move your body – take those stairs, do some housework and gardening, play with your kids.

By moving more in your everyday life you gain health benefits, become a little fitter and stronger and burn more calories – couple this with smart food choices and it will be enough to see you start to lose weight. Don't believe me? Just try it. Doing scheduled exercise is just a bonus for burning more calories, greater fitness gains and accelerating your weight loss. If moving more and eating smart sees you losing weight at first, what an easy way to make a start to The New You!

WORKSHOP: How can I be more active?

Here are some simple ways to move more. Circle or highlight any of the following activities you could apply to your everyday life and include more of your own examples.

- Clean the house – put some music on and clean faster.
- Vacuum.
- Scrub floors – use both arms and scrub in a circular motion, sideways and up and down for a great upper-body workout.

- Walk to the corner store for milk and the newspaper.
- Walk to deliver a message at work instead of emailing.
- Wash the car at the car wash.
- Do some gardening – weeding and digging are great for burning calories.
- Run and play with your kids.
- Hang out the clothes instead of using the dryer.
- Wash and dry the dishes instead of using the dishwasher.
- Take the stairs; if you already do, take them two at a time to burn more calories and work your backside.
- Get up and change the channel instead of using the remote.
- Do that home handy work you've been meaning to do.
- Take in the groceries one bag in each hand at a time (makes more trips).
- Park further away at the shopping centre and walk the difference.
- Go to a coffee shop that's further away than at the front door to the office.

Now add some more ideas of your own.

_____

_____

_____

_____

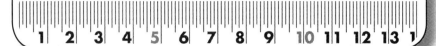

Of course, we know that we also need to exercise in addition to everyday activity, which brings us to the next step.

STEP 2 – To move more you need to exercise more

Doing more vigorous exercise than everyday activity provides the benefit of extra calorie burning and extra health benefits, such as extra protection against heart disease, and stress and depression management.

We all know we need to exercise more, but it's the 'doing' part that we struggle with. What stops us from doing it? Usually exercise excuses. The two most common ones are 'I don't have time' and 'I can't take time away from the kids'.

The hardest thing about exercise for most people is finding the time to do it, and for some people it really is a problem but not as big a problem as we make it out to be. There are simple ways around this challenge, and they are managing our time better and prioritising what is **most** important in our day.

Make it your priority
to find or make time to exercise
and take care of yourself.

If this means getting up a little earlier and going for a walk then so be it! How much do you want to lose weight? And remember it's only hard in the beginning. As you see results from exercise you will start to enjoy it more and then it will become easier to get yourself to do it. If I told you it would cost you a set price to lose weight and be healthy, I bet you, no matter what the cost, if it were guaranteed, you would do everything it takes to find the money. I am offering you a set price – only it doesn't cost anything other than some time and effort out of your day.

> *If you don't get up and do what needs to be done then regardless of how much you want it, it won't get done.*

It's all a matter of prioritising and organising. Stephen R Covey author of the bestselling book *The 7 Habits of Highly Effective People*, asks us to imagine you had a glass filled with some big stones. If you tried to fit another big rock in you would realise it won't fit, and would probably say 'The glass is full' and think there's nothing else you could do about it. What if the glass represented your day and the rocks are the things you have to get done. If you were to take smaller rocks and let them fall in around the big rocks you would fit more in. The glass is now full.

But if you were to take some even smaller pebbles and put them in the glass they would fall in around the big and little rocks. You have fit more stuff into the glass. The glass is now full.

But if you were to take some sand and pour it into the glass you would fit a lot more in. The glass is now full.

But if you were to pour some water into the glass, the glass would now be full. See how much more you can fit into your glass by organising (and prioritising) it all?

WORKSHOP: Scheduling exercise time

Draw seven columns and mark them Monday through to Sunday. Write down the time periods where you usually have to do something, such as work, bath the kids, cook dinner and so on. Then mark the time periods where you habitually do things that you don't have to do, such as 'veg' out in front of the TV, sleeping in and so on. Can you see where you might be able to make time to exercise?

The weekly planner you just did was your old day. Repeat this process and schedule in some time to exercise and do more physical activity. This one will be your new day – remember this is all about replacing your old ways of doing things that didn't work with new ways that do.

Another reason a lot of people cite for not exercising is because they don't want to be 'selfish' and they would rather spend the time with their loved ones. Let's take a moment to think about this. Say, hypothetically, you're obese and have children, and you want to spend all of your time with your kids. So you sit down with your kids and watch TV. In turn, your children follow the example set by you of spending family time being sedentary. They will also follow your lead in becoming obese.

> *Make sure that when your kids look up to you, they see what you want them to see.*

Conversely, imagine if you were 'selfish' and for, say, six to 12 months you took time out from them for an hour a day and spent that time working out and working on your health and weight, which in turn resulted in you having a greater self-esteem and a greater quality of life. Your children would follow the example you set by taking an interest in their health, working out, playing sports and participating in active family activities such as shooting hoops in the backyard and going for bike rides. They will also follow your lead in becoming healthy and happy, and develop a 'go get 'em', 'can-do' attitude.

Now tell me which one is less selfish?

That's just a little exercise to help you consider the fact that you may not be seeing the big picture: that changing your priorities is well worth it in the long run.

WORKSHOP: Exercise excuses

List the excuses you use for not exercising and offer some strategies to beat them.

Excuse: I'm too tired.
Excuse buster: I'll feel more energetic in general and get closer to my goals.

Excuse: What's the use?
Excuse buster: I am worth more than the effort I apply, and I know this.

Excuse: I can't afford a trainer, gym membership, workout gear and so on.
Excuse buster: I have joggers and a road outside ... that's enough.

Excuse: It hurts; I can't be bothered.
Excuse buster: I will hurt a whole lot more if I don't bother.

Excuse: I don't like it.
Excuse buster: Comfort never got me results; I need to get uncomfortable to get the results I want.

Excuse: I'm too busy.
Excuse buster: Too busy for what? If I don't have

time for me how will I ever have time to give my best to others?

(Now add some more of your own or add to the examples)

Excuse: _____

_____

_____

Excuse buster: _____

_____

_____

Excuse: _____

_____

_____

Excuse buster: _____

_____

_____

Excuse: _____

_____

_____

Excuse buster: _____

_____

_____

1 2 3 4 5 6 7 8 9 10 11 12 13 1

Now that we have got the exercise excuses out of the way, let's look at the best ways to exercise. The best place to get started with some exercise and a more active lifestyle is walking.

STEP 3 – To move more, you need to simply walk more

Why walking? Walking is simple to do, it costs nothing and you can do it right now by stepping out your front door, plus it is not too strenuous but it has a high enough impact on your activity levels that you will start to see results fairly quickly. Start from today and make walking as much of a habit as brushing your teeth. Whether you walk for exercise or to be more active (keep in mind, if you're walking for exercise, a leisurely doing-the-groceries type of walk just won't cut it; you need to walk at a reasonable pace where you can feel the walk – in either your leg muscles or your breathing). In the workshop on the following page, you can find some suggestions for fitting walking into your day.

> *TIP*   Studies show that dog owners do more walking and suffer less stress and depression than non dog owners.

WORKSHOP: How can I fit more walking into my day?

- Walk the dog – if you don't have one volunteer at your local shelter, adopt a dog, offer to walk the neighbour's dog or start a dog-walking business for extra cash.
- Walk the kids to and from school.
- Walk either to and from the bus stop or to and from work.
- Get on or off the bus or train one–two stops earlier or later and walk.
- Use walking as your preferred mode of transport.
- Walk to do the groceries and then get them home delivered.
- Find a walking friend, or make walking the time when you and your partner can bond and discuss the day's events.

Add some more of your own ideas or highlight any of the above suggestions that you could implement, and then mark them in your diary or weekly planner.

1 2 3 4 5 6 7 8 9 10 11 12 13 1

And there is another thing we have to factor in to our exercise equation – resistance training.

STEP 4 – To move more you need to lift more

Resistance training simply means lifting a resistance and this resistance can come in many forms such as:

- Using the weight of another person, for example, piggybacking someone while you do squats or push-ups, piggybacking your kids, carrying a baby or small toddler.
- Carrying heavy items around your house and yard, such as shovelling dirt and lifting boxes, even taking in the groceries and lifting items such as bags of flour or tins of food.
- Lifting your own body weight, such as doing push-ups and sit-ups.
- Using free weights, such as dumbbells, barbells or medicine balls.
- Working out with machine weights in a gym.
- Using a resistance band.
- Doing a circuit.

Resistance training helps maintain your metabolism; builds bone strength, which is great for helping prevent osteoporosis; firms flabby bits such as bottoms and arms; and burns calories, especially when done in a circuit style.

WORKSHOP: Tips to help you move more

- **Do some circuit training:** Circuit training is my favourite! It simply means moving from one exercise to another with little to no rest. It's great for variety, combining resistance and cardio benefits into the one workout and for burning loads of calories.

- **Remind yourself why you want to exercise:** Exercise is so good for the body, mind and soul so get on up and move. Anytime is always a good time to do something.

- **Challenge yourself:** One of the biggest mistakes people make when exercising for weight loss is not working hard enough by forgetting to progress the intensity of the workout.

  A little healthy competition, with yourself or another, will push you to reach your true potential. Sooner or later you will have to challenge yourself because your once hard workout will become easy and if you don't up the ante you won't keep getting results. For example, walk faster or further; lift more weight; work your way up to running; do more of the exercises you don't really like (these are normally the ones that are hardest for you!); or hire a personal trainer to push you to new limits – if one-on-one personal training is not affordable, group personal training is much cheaper, sharing the cost between two or more people. To find a qualified trainer near you go to *www.fitness.org.au*

continued

- **Mix things up:** Two of the biggest factors for dropping out of an exercise program are boredom and not seeing the results of your hard work. Mix things up by trying a different exercise, a new workout or exercise class such as cycle, boxing and aerobics classes; walking or running on different surfaces such as the beach and bush; training for a fun run; starting a sport; training at different times of the day; getting a training partner; joining a walking or running group. The options are endless, just keep searching and trying new things that maintain your interest.

- **The more you put into exercise, the more you get out of it:** There are many factors that come into the exercise part of the weight loss equation, from just getting out there and moving right through to specific exercise planning and programming and seeing professional trainers. It is all beneficial, but what you sow you reap, and the more effort you make to move as much as possible and exercise as hard as you can will determine how quickly you get results.

- **Limit sitting time:** Try to limit the amount of spare time you have being sedentary: don't sit still, don't sit in front of the TV on the lounge, or if you're going to watch TV, set up some cardio equipment such as a treadmill, stationary bike or stepper (if you don't have one collecting dust in the garage, you can buy or rent one, see *www.workoutworld. com.au*) and use it during your TV viewing times.

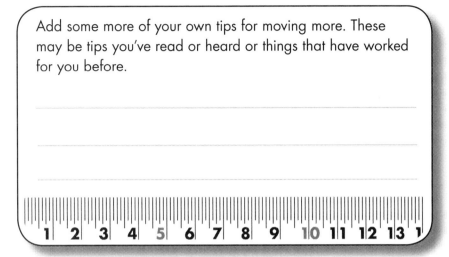

Add some more of your own tips for moving more. These may be tips you've read or heard or things that have worked for you before.

Achievements so far

Congratulations, you are now being completely honest with yourself about your motives and reasons for weight loss plus you will have learnt how to 'Move More'. With this part I hope you have:

✔ Discovered simple ways to move more and come up with your own ideas to be more active each day.

✔ Drawn up a weekly schedule and written down the time periods where you are busy doing things you have to do (such as work, cooking dinner, etc). Then written down the times where you have breaks in your schedule (such as sleeping in, watching TV, etc), then organised your time to fit in exercise.

✔ Listed the excuses you use for not exercising and have come up with your own positive strategies to beat them.

✔ Found ways to fit more walking into your day.

✔ Created your own 'Move More' tips to help target your weight loss.

THE NEW ~~ME~~ YOU

Where are you up to?

WEEK: **WEIGHT:**

Emotional state ....

....

Physical state ....

....

Challenges ....

....

Accomplishments ....

....

POSITIVE PLUS:

I feel great today because ....

I am amazing because ....

I will/am succeed/ing because ....

GOALS:

INSPIRATIONAL QUOTE:

THINK THIN

You may have started to lose weight, but find yourself with the same mindset as a fat person (just as I did). You may still have low self-esteem, be avoiding social situations or just not believing you're worth it. You need to make sure your mind changes along with your weight as your thoughts and emotions may hold you back from continuing to lose weight or even be one of the causes of the yo-yo effect of dieting. You need to think like a slim person. For example, if you're trying to give up smoking and keep telling yourself you have to quit, you'll probably try countless times but never be able to kick the habit; if you see yourself as a non-smoker – feeling healthy, breathing easy, being able to run up a set of stairs, more attractive because you no longer reek of cigarette smoke and so on – you will be able to give up. In other words, a smoker will give up when they see themselves as a non-smoker, not a smoker who is quitting; an overweight person will be able to lose weight and live slim when they see themselves as a slim person, not as an overweight person who is trying to lose weight.

So how do we get ourselves to **think thin**? Thinking thin takes work. It's not a habit that you have, because you are used to thinking like a fat person (with 'fattitude', as coined by author Craig Harper in his book of the same name), which means your head is probably full of put-downs, self-hating and self-critical thoughts. Just like you have to learn how to Eat Smart and Move More, you have to learn how to Think Thin – this means thinking positive and with self-love.

One of the best ways to start monitoring your thoughts and feelings is to keep a journal. You might like to go out and buy yourself a special journal, perhaps with an inspiring picture or design printed on the cover or one with inspiring quotes printed on the pages – make this something special that's just for you. Or you can use one of the 'Think Thin Journals' in Part 4: The New Me Tool Kit. This will be your very own private space to reflect and focus on what's positive in your life and about you.

You can use your journal to record anything that comes to mind about your weight loss and inner journey. I strongly encourage you to write down only positive things about your life and self because what we focus on expands. If we're always focusing on the negative it becomes a magnet for attracting more negative energy. This is about creating a New You and a new way of thinking.

WORKSHOP: Positive reinforcement

Write down some positive things about yourself right now. (This cannot be something negative with a positive spin on it, such as 'I went for a walk today, but I gave up halfway and turned around to come back'. It can only be positive, such as 'I motivated myself to get out for a short walk today!')

_____

_____

_____

_____

_____

| 1 | 2 | 3 | 4 | 5 | 6 | 7 | 8 | 9 | 10 | 11 | 12 | 13 | 1 |

Getting negative thoughts out of your head and on to paper is helpful; sometimes just seeing your thoughts written down shows you how silly and self-defeating they are. The first step towards thinking thin is monitoring your self-talk, and replacing negative talk with positive talk.

STEP 1 – To think thin you need to think positive

Just like ridding your kitchen of trigger foods, you need to rid your brain of negative thoughts.

We can only fit so much stuff inside of us – if we're full of negativity then there isn't any room for the positive.

You need to become your own support network. What kinds of supportive words would you offer to a friend if they spoke one of your negative thoughts out loud to you? This is the way you have to treat yourself: with kindness and compassion, gently encouraging your thoughts into affirming, positive thoughts. Even if you don't buy into what you say yet, you will. It's a case of fake it until you make it.

If you hear something enough times, you will believe it.

WORKSHOP: Changing your thoughts

List some of your negative self-talk and replace each thought with a more positive, affirming thought.

Negative: I've failed before, it won't be any different this time.

Positive: The reason it will be different this time is because I will do different things to what I usually do, and this will help me stick to it.

Negative: It's so hard to lose weight.

Positive: I will feel better and it will get easier to lose as I lose more weight.

Negative: I don't deserve to be happy.

Positive: I deserve to be happy just as much as the next person; if I am happy then my happiness will spill over to others and, in turn, I can make many people happy.

Negative: I'm safe being fat.

Positive: Being healthy and happy makes me safe.

Negative: What's the point, I may as well just accept this is the way I am?

Positive: I will not give up on myself.

Negative: No one believes in me.

Positive: I believe in me.

Negative: I'm constantly losing this weight battle.

Positive: If I arm myself with the correct weapons and attitude I will win.

Negative: I have no control.

Positive: I am in control (over everything I choose to do and be).

Add some more of your own:

Negative:

Positive:

Negative:

Positive:

Negative:

Positive:

Negative:

Positive:

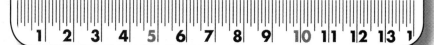

To really help you understand the true nature of negative self-talk, you need to tap into that negative person lurking within your subconscious. It helps to name the person who speaks so negatively to you (for me it was Mr Negativity) to bring this person to the surface. Every time you catch yourself using negative self-talk put it back onto someone; make it come from someone you can address.

WORKSHOP: Q & A

Now that you have named your negative self, ask yourself a few questions, and then answer them:

Would you put up with or accept what this person (your negative self) is saying to you from someone else?

Would you allow your friends or someone in your life to speak to you like that?

If they did, what would you do about it?

Why not do this with your negative self?

What actions would you take to remove this negative person from your life?

Once you work on this process and get rid of enough of the negatives and replace them with positives, you end up at a point where you don't need to work hard or put effort in to have the positive in your life. It will happen automatically.

Now that you're thinking more positively, you will need to create positive images to match your positive thoughts.

STEP 2 – To think thin you need to visualise yourself as thin

The best way to do this is through visualisation. Visualisation is a tool used by all successful people; they see and feel themselves being successful – crossing the finish line first, standing on the dais accepting their medal, getting that job promotion – long before their actual success. This is the process of creating memories that haven't yet happened. You set the image up, hone your focus which is like tuning into a frequency, and align your energy until you manifest your memory. This is called the law of attraction. (I'm sure you've heard about *The Secret, www.thesecret.tv*). Create a mind map, make a poster or a collage of words and images to inspire you and guide you towards your goal. Try using your face on any body images you use.

*Create positive images to match
your positive thoughts.*

WORKSHOP: Visualise a New You

Where would you like to be, what would you like to look and feel like, and what would you like to be doing in?

1 month:

_____

_____

_____

12 months:

_____

_____

_____

5 years:

_____

_____

_____

10 years:

_____

_____

1 2 3 4 5 6 7 8 9 10 11 12 13 1

However, seeing and feeling yourself as slim and successful is not enough. You need to believe you have the ability to do this.

STEP 3 – To think thin you need to believe in yourself

You manifest what you believe you deserve. See it, feel it, believe it and you will create it – this is called manifestation.

You have the power to do this, and anything you set your mind to; actually you have already done this and succeeded, you just need to make sure you hang around long enough to see that.

Your negative self always tells you that you can't, and you usually buy into it and believe you can't. It's time to stand up for yourself and affirm that you can! It's time to find your self-belief.

WORKSHOP: Believing that you can lose weight

List as many reasons, if any, as you can think of, as to why you don't believe you can lose weight and get healthy:

Now, list 10 reasons why you believe you can lose weight and get healthy:

1.
2.
3.
4.
5.
6.
7.
8.
9.
10.

Last, but definitely not least, you need to practise self-love.

STEP 4 – To think thin you need to love yourself

So many of us go through our lives carrying such self-loathing and self-hatred around. The energy you send out is the energy you get back. If you want others to love you, love yourself. If you want others to believe in you, love yourself enough to believe in yourself. If you want others to support you in your weight loss journey, love yourself enough to support yourself. Also, more often than not, our outer obesity is merely a symptom of our inner inability to love ourselves and be true to ourselves. All health and happiness starts with being authentic and loving and honouring your true self. (So go out and buy yourself a little rose quartz, which is known for love and healing the heart.)

Losing weight and gaining health is the ultimate act of self-love.

WORKSHOP: Tips for thinking thin

- **Surround yourself with people who think thin:**
Like attracts like, which means that if you want to be at
the top of the world then hang around people who are
at the top of the world; if you want to be fit and healthy
don't hang around couch potatoes and people who aren't
active. (If you can't avoid it because your family isn't
willing to change with you, that's okay, you can make
positive friendships.) We subconsciously become products
of our environments, so consciously create the environment
you wish to become a product of.

- **Get support from people who think and act
positive:** When things get tough, and they will because
it's part of life, be sure to have a support system of positive
people around you who can uplift you, encourage you
and remind you of why losing weight is important to you.
Remember that story of the footprints in the sand: a man
asks God when reflecting on his life why at certain times he
sees only one set of footprints, and he thinks God left him
to walk alone when things got tough. God answers, 'I didn't
leave you, the set of footprints you see are mine, I was
carrying you.' What an awesome concept.

- **Trust yourself:** When you hear yourself say, 'Oh, I
shouldn't eat that?' or 'I should exercise', listen to yourself.
Don't let it slide, forget you said it or even tell yourself to
shut up. It is really important to listen to your positive self
and make sure that you follow through with the things you
know you should be doing rather than doing the things
you shouldn't be doing because they're easier.

continued

- **Meditate:** Meditation helps you stay calm and connect with your true self. Meditation doesn't have to see you sit cross-legged and light incense. It can be anything that allows you to find some stillness – perhaps it's walking in nature, doing yoga, listening to a meditation tape, or simply sitting under a tree.

- **Stay present:** We all often miss the present because we are so busy worrying about the past and stressing about the future. This is counterproductive to your well-being and also your weight because stress is a known cause of weight gain, particularly around the stomach. It doesn't matter where you've been or how far you have to go, what matters is just doing your best. For a great source on practising the power of now, visit *www.eckharttolle.com*.

- **Use affirmations:** Affirmations (positive sayings or rules) are a brilliant reminder of what it is that you want or need in your life, and help you to create the outcomes you truly want.

WORKSHOP: I am

Create your own personal affirmation or mantra, something you can repeat to yourself every day and every time you feel like giving up, such as, 'I am beautiful, I believe in myself, I will succeed at everything I try and I am worth so much more than the effort I am putting in right now.'

My mantra is:

Achievements so far

Congratulations, you have now been completely honest with yourself about your motives and reasons for weight loss plus you will have learnt how to 'Think Thin'. With this part I hope you have:

✔ Written down positive things about yourself in your special 'Positive Journal'.

✔ Listed some of your negative self-talk and replaced each thought with a more positive, affirming thought.

✔ Named your negative self and asked it questions and then answered these questions.

✔ Worked out where you would like to be, look like and feel like and started the process of manifestation

✔ Listed reasons as to why you don't believe you can lose weight and get healthy and then counteracted these with at least ten reasons why you believe you can lose weight and get healthy.

I'd like to take this opportunity to congratulate you on getting this far. If you have read through the book and completed the worksheets (if you haven't then go back and do any you have missed) you have proven you really want the results. You have prepared yourself to Eat Smart, Move More and Think Thin, and laid down the solid foundations necessary to begin building The New You.

THE NEW ~~ME~~ YOU

Where are you up to?

WEEK: WEIGHT:

Emotional state _____

_____

Physical state _____

_____

Challenges _____

_____

Accomplishments _____

_____

POSITIVE PLUS:

I feel great today because _____

I am amazing because _____

I will/am succeed/ing because _____

GOALS:

INSPIRATIONAL QUOTE:

PART 4

The New Me Tool Kit

Putting the program into practice to build The New You

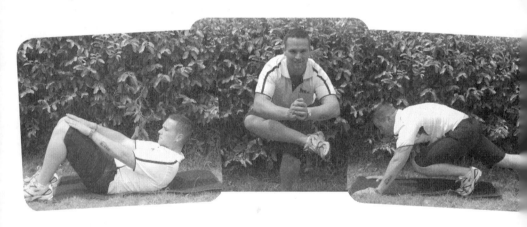

LEFT TO RIGHT: and **OPPOSITE:** Me in training mode at The New Me Weight Loss Retreat. You don't need to go to a gym to work out, there are more than enough places in your everyday life that can be used for free. Here I am in the garden at my retreat.

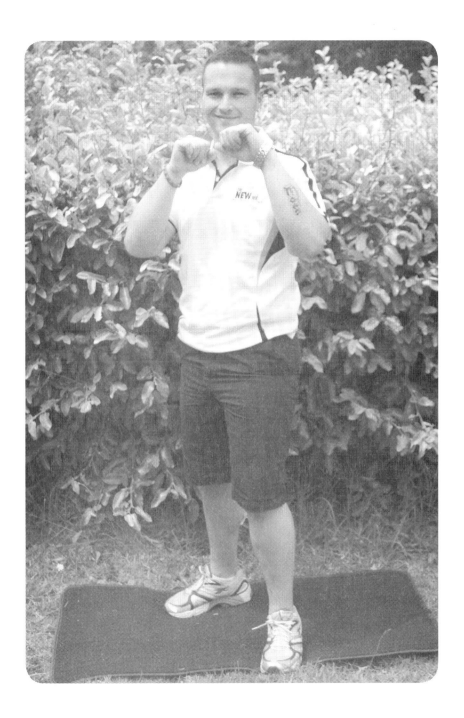

The New Me Program is based on the three key principles: Eat Smart, Move More, Think Thin. You have just learnt all about these principles in Part 3 and now it is time to put your work into practice. This part provides you with the tool kit you need to build a new body, a new life and a New You!

Grab that pen or pencil again. You have to do a bit of calculating, some more homework and journaling but this is going to help you devise the perfect eating and exercise plan for you and your weight loss goals. This is all about putting time into You. Starting now. Dedicate yourself and get ready to discover a New You.

I'm about to give you all the hands-on, practical tools you need to build The New You, but before we embark on this life-changing journey together, there are three things I need to say to you.

1. *You have the ability to do this, no matter how many times you have tried before – anything is achievable.*

2. *You can consciously decide and control the process of losing weight.*

3. *I may be giving you the tools, but it is up to you to put into practice what you will learn and have learnt up to now in this book.*

Counting and calculating calories

To make sure you're on the right track with your diet and exercise and weight loss program, you need to: firstly, start counting calories, and secondly, understand calories. Before you baulk at the thought of being a slave to calorie counting your whole life, counting calories and calculating equations is simply a short-term process aimed at raising your awareness about your food choices (quite often we don't realise just how many calories we're consuming until we take the time to look), and the necessary balance between exercise and food needed to achieve weight loss.

To help make the process of counting and calculating calories a lot easier, I recommend you get yourself two things:

1. **A caloric counting book**. You can find the amount of calories contained in foods through the internet but it's handy to have a pocket book to keep with you at all times so you can check things as you eat them. The best source is the Calorie King website *www.calorieking.com.au* and *Allan Borushek's Pocket Calorie, Fat & Carbohydrate Counter*, which is revised each year and costs around $10. This is also available to buy from my website, *www.thenewme.com.au* Don't worry, before long you will know what foods carry too many calories and you will be able to choose the best foods without even thinking about it or checking in with a calorie counter.

2. **A heart rate monitor that calculates calories**. Look for one that calculates the calories you burn through your exercise and activity, as well as the total amount of calories you expend each day (Total Daily Energy Expenditure TDEE – more on this later). There are some well-priced simple units

on the market, and if you can't afford one you can still do the calculating yourself using formulas and a calculator and pen and paper, or through an online calculator – there are many out there, so do a search. As you can imagine, though, all this calculating can be time consuming, which is why a heart rate monitor that does the calculating for you is so handy and something to work towards getting – perhaps you can make it your next Christmas, birthday, Easter or anniversary gift to yourself. You can purchase a heart rate monitor through your local exercise equipment store, some pharmacies, some gyms, through catalogues via the mail or internet, or through my website, *www.thenewme.com.au*

So why does calculating calories matter? The energy equation (calories in versus calories out). **Put more calories in than you put out and you gain weight; put less calories in than you put out and you lose weight; put the same amount of calories in as you put out and you maintain your weight.** 'Calories in' come from the foods we eat and the drinks we drink; 'calories out' comes from the energy we burn up through our basic daily movements, metabolism and exercise.

While this formula of weight gain and loss is simple, don't be fooled into thinking that weight loss is always a simple case of mathematics. The physiological reason for gaining weight is pretty simple – basic sedentariness and substance abuse (the substance being food) – but the reasons we find it hard to lose weight aren't always so simple and methodical; for example, there could be mental or emotional reasons behind your weight loss struggle, which is what we address in the Think Thin part of The New Me Program back in Part 3: The New Me Program.

But, for most of us, if we use or burn up more calories than we put into our body, and create what is called a calorie deficit, then we will most likely lose weight (so long as the calories in aren't rubbish).

Calculating calorie deficits

How do we make this deficit? Your TDEE comes from the amount of energy you expend through physical activity and exercise as well as your Basal Metabolic Rate (BMR), also called Resting Metabolic Rate (RMR). Your BMR is basically the rate or amount of calories your body burns in a day at rest, meaning that if you didn't do anything active all day your body would still burn a certain amount of calories just to stay alive. Your BMR accounts for around 60 to 70 per cent of the energy you expend each day. This is interesting for you to know – that just as your body is now, you're burning calories, and if you simply added the right foods and ate less than what your body is burning, you would start losing weight, even without exercising. The weight loss would be slow because the deficit wouldn't be that big, but it would still start to happen. What an inspiring place to start. **Right here, right now, if you eat smarter, you will start seeing results immediately!**

You can calculate your BMR using an online BMR calculator, (see *www.thenewme.com.au*). Or, you can work it out now, using the following Mifflin calculation:

Men: (10 x weight in kg) + (6.25 x height in cm)
– (5 x age) + 5 = BMR in calories
Women: (10 x weight in kg) + (6.25 x height in cm)
– (5 x age) – 161 = BMR in calories

For example, if you're a 40-year-old female who weighs 140 kilograms and you're 170 centimetres tall, your BMR would be: 2102 calories. So if this female ate less calories than this, she would make a calorie deficit, and she would start to lose weight. And if she exercised on top of this, she would make even more of a deficit and lose even more.

WORKSHOP: Calculate your BMR

Using the Mifflin calculation, work out your BMR. Write down your BMR in a weight loss journal to keep a record of it to help with further calculations. Your BMR equals ....

So how much of a deficit do you need to make to lose weight?

Scientists have worked out from the average BMR that it takes a deficit of 7700 calories to lose 1 kilogram (2.2 pounds) of weight. So a standard prescription to follow is to make an 1100-calorie deficit each day to lose 1 kilogram (2.2 pounds) a week. However, if you make this deficit – providing you do it safely by maintaining a balanced diet and exercising – in less than a week you should, theoretically, lose more than 1 kilogram (2.2 pounds) a week.

So whether you take five, seven or 10 days to make your deficit will depend on the time you have available to train and prepare low-calorie meals, as well as how well you're able to handle temptations that pop up.

To sum up, the rate at which you make your deficit will determine the speed in which your weight loss occurs. The basic mathematics behind this formula looks like this:

Calories out (BMR + Physical Activity and Exercise) –
Calories in (Food + Drink) = Calorie Deficit (CD)

(CD + CD + CD + CD + CD + CD +CD) = Total Calorie Deficit per week (TCDPW)

TCDPW divided by 7700 = kilograms/pounds lost that week

So now let's take more of a look at the left side of the equation 'Calories out' and 'Calories in'.

Counting calories in and out

So we now know that the 'calorie in' part of the equation is the amount of calories you eat and drink; and the 'calorie out' part of the equation is the total amount of energy you expend each day (TDEE), and this comes from your BMR as well as the physical activity you do, so someone who is more active will expend more energy each day than someone who is less active. Got it? Therefore your activity levels need to be taken into account to get a more accurate indication of the right calorie deficit for you. Again, you can do this through an online calculator, or use the formula below.

- **If you lead a sedentary lifestyle** (little or no exercise, desk job) = **BMR x 1.2**
- **If you are only lightly active** (light exercise/sports 1–3 days/week) = **BMR x 1.375**
- **If you are moderately active** (moderate exercise/sports 3–5 days/week) = **BMR x 1.55**
- **If you are very active** (hard exercise/sports 6–7 days/week) = **BMR x 1.725**
- **If you are extremely active** (hard daily exercise/sports and physical job or 2 training sessions a day training) = **BMR x 1.9**

So using our previous example of the female with a BMR of 2102 calories, if she led a sedentary lifestyle, she would multiply her BMR by 1.2, and her TDEE would be 2522 calories; but if she was to take up a little walking, she would be lightly active, so she would multiply her BMR by 1.375, and her TDEE would now be 2890 calories.

> Using the calculation above and your BMR from the previous calculation, work out your level of activity, and work out your TDEE. _____

Now going back to the CD formula, and following on with our example, if she ate 1200 calories a day and did the same amount of exercise every day for seven days, her daily calorie deficit would be 1690 calories; her TCDPW would be 11830 calories; and her estimated weight loss would be 1.54 kilograms (3.4 pounds) per week.

> Using the CD formula and your TDEE from the previous calculation, assuming you went on a 1200-calorie per day diet, work out your estimated weekly weight loss. (Now this should get you excited! And remember if you add more exercise you will lose even more weight!) _____
>
> _____

A more accurate way is to use the sedentary calculation (BMR x 1.2), and add the calories burned through physical activity and exercise on top of this. This is how I would like you to log your calorie output each day in your Food and Exercise Diary.

Multiply your BMR by 1.2, and keep this number handy, so you can put it into your Food and Exercise Diary every day, adding calories burned through activity and exercise on top of this number: My BMR (...................) x 1.2 = ...

To work out how many calories you burn through exercise and activity, look it up on the internet, or use the chart below, which provides an estimated number of calories expended at various body weights for typical exercise and activities done for 30 minutes. Please note: The figures below are provided as estimates only.

Exercise and activity calorie chart

This table provides a general glance at the average calories burned in 30 minutes for common forms of exercise, activity and incidental activity.

EXERCISE AND ACTIVITY	CALORIES BURNED PER 30 MIN		
	70 kg	100 kg	150 kg
Aerobics (low impact)	178	254	380
Basketball (leisurely)	201	287	430
Ten-pin bowling	85	121	182
Canoeing/rowing (light effort)	108	154	231
Canoeing/rowing (moderate effort)	209	298	446
Circuit training (moderate–vigorous effort/ aerobic and weight-lifting exercises)	393	562	843
Cycling (light effort)	193	276	413
Cycling (moderate effort)	309	441	661

EXERCISE AND ACTIVITY	CALORIES BURNED PER 30 MIN		
Dancing (general)	154	220	331
Dancing (slow)	85	121	182
Gardening (general)	88	126	189
Gardening (digging)	240	343	514
Golfing (walking w/o cart, pulling clubs)	154	220	331
Golfing (with a cart)	108	154	231
Hiking	240	342	513
Ironing	88	126	189
Jogging (general)	286	408	612
Pilates	150	214	321
Playing frisbee	105	150	225
Playing (including spurts of walking/ running) with children	140	200	300
Mowing lawn	193	276	414
Running (general)	355	507	761
Scrubbing floors on hands and knees	193	276	414
Sex	135	193	289
Shopping	75	107	160
Skipping rope (general)	440	628	942
Soccer (casual/general)	301	430	645
Spinning (cycle class)	375	536	804
Squash	316	452	678
Stair climber machine	247	353	529
Stair climbing (walking upstairs)	216	309	463

EXERCISE AND ACTIVITY	CALORIES BURNED PER 30 MIN		
Sweeping floors	140	200	300
Swimming (general)	186	265	397
Tennis (general)	247	353	529
Vacuuming	150	214	321
Walking (slow pace)	92	132	198
Walking (moderate pace)	123	176	265
Walking (brisk pace)	154	220	331
Walking dog	123	176	264
Washing car	150	214	321
Washing dishes	52	74	111
Weight training (moderate to vigorous effort)	291	419	628
Weight training (light effort)	193	276	413
Yoga	141	201	301

Note: Calories burnt vary according to age, sex, muscle mass, fitness levels and weight. Figures based on averages. If you do the activity for an hour, simply double the calorie expenditure for your closest weight. If you want to calculate for the precise amount of minutes you spent on doing an activity, simply divide the calorie amount for your closest weight by 30 to get calorie expenditure per minute and then multiply it by the minutes you spent doing the activity. For example, if you walked at a brisk pace for 40 minutes and you weigh 90 kilograms you would use the 100-kilogram column: Walking (brisk pace) burns 220 calories for 30 minutes; 220/30 = 7.3; 7.3 x 40 (minutes) = 293 calories burned in 40 minutes.

Use the Exercise and Activity Calorie Chart and your calorie-counting book to log your calorie intake and output and calculate your deficit. You can log all of this into the Food and Exercise Diary on pages 244–5, or you can simply make your own using a notebook or computer template.

Don't forget, you can make it even easier by using a heart rate monitor, or online calculator, such as the Calorie King Nutrition and Exercise Manager, *www.calorieking.com.au*

Okay, so now that we have learnt what it is we are trying to achieve let's look at how we can work on getting this to happen, starting with eating smart.

EAT SMART DIET

The menu plans are based on the diet plan I followed, and still follow today, which allowed me to shed over 50 kilograms (110 pounds) in four months, and has allowed me to keep the weight off ever since. This is also the eating program offered at The New Me Weight Loss Retreat. It is called the Eat Smart Diet and is a **high-protein, low-carbohydrate, low-fat, low-calorie** way of eating.

Some of the benefits of eating this way are:

- High-protein diets help to stabilise blood sugar and curb cravings.

- Many successful well-known diet plans are based on the protein principle and have a proven track record of getting results.

- Protein helps to fill you up and usually takes less calories to do so than carbohydrates.

- Eating protein burns calories; your body has to work harder to digest protein than it does carbohydrates.

- Eating large doses of carbohydrates causes influxes of insulin, which is known to stimulate appetite, promote fat storage and prevent fat from being released for energy; too much insulin in the body can, over time, lead to insulin resistance, which is a precursor to Type 2 diabetes.

- Adequate protein is necessary for muscle growth, and for recovery and repair from exercise.

- Excess carbohydrates that are not utilised by the body end up being stored as fat.

- Keeping your fat content low helps you to keep your calorie content low, because fat is calorie dense.

- Keeping calories low ensures that you create a greater deficit enabling more-rapid weight loss results.

- Extensive research has found that low-calorie diets can offer health benefits and increase life expectancy.

For a **short while** I find it very beneficial to drop major carbohydrates, both simple and complex such as **bread, pasta, sugary vegetables (such as potato, pumpkin, carrot, corn, peas and beans) and fruit.**

Although fruit is obviously really good for you – it's packed with vitamins and fibre (fibre slows down the absorption of the sugars from fruit) – it's still a form of sugar. Initially, you need to focus on reducing all of the sugar in your body, so this is the reason for excluding fruit from your diet at first. Quite often the first thing people do when going on a diet is to overdose on fruit because it's 'healthy' meaning you often end up adding more sugar to your already sugar-loaded body, making it even harder to get off on the right foot. Eliminating all sugars, including fruit, for a short period of time allows your body to:

- Cleanse.

- Enter a state of ketosis – you would be familiar with this term from popular no-carb diets – which forces your body to utilise energy from its fat stores rather than its first preference for energy, sugar (glucose), because there is none readily available. (If you really want to know if you're in a state of ketosis, you can check this with special urine test strips, such as 'ketostix'.)

- Retrain your taste buds to receive enough sweet satisfaction from a piece of fruit, which is hardly breaking one's diet, once you reintroduce fruit.

If you do decide to cut out fruit, I only recommend doing this for the purpose of a cleanse for no more than 1–2 days. **For longer periods of fruit restriction, lasting more than 1–2 days, please do so under supervision (check with a dietitian or doctor) and take a fruit and vegetable supplement.**

Diet guidelines

- *How many calories?*

I recommend **1200–1300 calories per day for a male** and around **1000–1200 calories per day for a female.**

Note: This is a relatively low calorie amount, however, I can say that you will not only survive on this amount of calories each day but it will ensure you lose weight at a fast-enough pace. You don't have to jump to this amount straightaway, especially if you're obese or morbidly obese; you can work your way down to this calorie quota, and before following a diet of this calorie amount, you must check with a doctor. Remember that protein helps you to feel full.

- ## What can I drink?

While water is the preference for making up your daily fluid quota, if you want to include other drinks, as long as they're water-based or diet drinks, that's fine, for example diet cordial or soft drink, herbal tea and small amounts of black tea with non-fat milk and no sugar or sugar replacer. Coffee or caffeinated soft drinks don't count towards your fluid quota as they dehydrate you.

- ## What about alcohol?

Alcoholic drinks contain sugar and calories, and when you drink alcohol the body has no place to store it, meaning your body will burn off the alcohol as its first preference and your fat stores don't get as much of a chance to be burned up. Alcohol also hinders your weight loss by the carefree (greasy!) food choices you tend to make when drunk and/or hung-over. If you do choose to have alcohol, aim for low-calorie options such as low- or no carb beer or vodka with soda water and a piece of fresh lime (not lime cordial which has sugar and calories) – but remember, the more obstacles you put in your path the longer it will take you to reach your goals and the bumpier the ride will be.

- ## How much fat?

Keep fats to a minimum: use only healthy fats such as olive oil and oil spray, foods such as avocados or nuts and choose very lean cuts of meat. Don't eat anything with more than 5–10 grams of fat per 100 grams, and keep an eye on the calorie content.

- ## What about eating out?

For the first 1–2 weeks, it's best to avoid eating out, so you know you're not getting excess fat and calories you didn't plan for. Then, you can decide whether you want to reintroduce meals that involve eating out (you can find tips for eating out on pages 188–93).

• *Should I take supplements?*

I recommend taking a good multi-vitamin and mineral supplement just to be sure you're not missing out on important nutrients while you're learning how to eat them all through your food without blowing out in calorie consumption. If you can't stomach dairy, simply replace with fortified soy products (calcium is not naturally found in soymilk so it must be added in), or be sure to take a calcium supplement. And, if you're going to practise a period of fruit restriction, supplement with a fruit and vegetable extract replacement. **Note:** High-protein, low-carbohydrate diets can cause constipation, so prunes have been added to the diet plan. In addition to this, keep up your water intake, take a fibre supplement if necessary or sprinkle some psyllium husks on your food or in your drinks. Simply ask your doctor, dietitian, local pharmacist or health food store for the best supplements to suit your requirements. Or, you can purchase organic supplements through my site, *www.thenewme.com.au*

• *Cleanse*

Before you start your diet, when you find your weight loss is stalling, or when you just can't get past constant cravings, I suggest cleansing for 1–2 days, by eating just protein – the easiest way is to use protein shakes and prepared cleanses available from pharmacies and health food stores or, just eat lean chicken and egg whites. I suggest no more than two days on the shakes, though, because you don't want to get sick of being on them or become reliant – remember the goal is to find a way of eating smart that will keep you slim forever, and drinking shakes forever wouldn't be smart because you'd get very bored!

Cleansing helps you to:

1. Prepare yourself for the new way of eating.

2. Give your body a shock so it responds better to the change.

3. Enhance your appreciation of healthy food because you have had two days without variety, as opposed to going from normal unlimited bad food to limited diet food and perhaps you're feeling resentful about it.

• *Adjust the diet to suit you*

You have all of the flexibility you need to mix and match meals (space has been provided for you to do this in the Make-Your-Own Menu Plan on pages 182–4), just make sure you stick to the suggested calorie limit and you eat a nutritious diet. If you find, when getting into your new style of eating, that something just isn't working for you, simply change that part of the diet. For example, I ate a lot of fish as part of my diet, but you may hate seafood, so what you need to do is find a replacement for this such as lean meat or grilled chicken. Or perhaps you live in a family where your diet is based around your native food, so a diet that factors in the types of foods the family eats will be more practical for you. **Remember:**

- **The more work you put into making a diet your own, something that really suits you, the better chance you're giving yourself to be able to stick with it long term.**

- **Don't beat up on yourself for not being able to stick to a diet plan; just learn from it, rectify it, make changes to the diet plan if necessary, and keep moving forward!**

Menu plans

In this section you will find three menu plans:

1. 7-Day Menu Plan

2. Make-Your-Own Menu Plan

3. Maintenance Menu Plan

The 7-Day Menu Plan is designed to kickstart your weight loss, and would ideally be followed for 1–4 weeks before moving onto the Make-Your-Own Menu Plan (or if you're happy to keep going with the 7-Day Menu Plan, you can), which you would follow until you reach your goal weight, at which point you would move onto the Maintenance Menu Plan.

Preparing for the 7-Day Menu Plan

Here's the 7-Day Menu Plan at a glance:

- 1200–1300 calories per day for a male and around 1000–1200 calories per day for a female, based on the following calorie breakdown:

  Breakfast: around 200 calories

  Lunch and dinner: around 300 calories per meal

  Snacks: around 100 calories per snack (minimum of two snacks, maximum of four snacks)

- If you're obese or morbidly obese, you may add 100 extra calories per meal and work your way down to the suggested calorie quota at your own pace. Remember, protein has a high satiety factor so you will feel fuller from eating less calories than you are used to.

- Snacks are to be eaten in between meals. Include a minimum of two snacks and a maximum of four snacks.
- Drink at least eight glasses of water a day plus an extra 1–2 for every hour of exercise.
- Everything must be lean, no excess fat.
- No fruit (fresh, dried or juice) except the allowed prunes. (Only when restricting fruit. Don't forget to check with a doctor or health professional before doing this.)
- No starchy or complex carbohydrates, unless necessary (see Note on page 172). Add carbohydrates if required from the middle column in the 'Allowed food groups' list on pages 171–2.
- No sugar (if needed, use artificial sweetener).
- No oils, except oil spray.

Here's a sample list of allowed food groups. These are just some of the basic foods you can eat, put into categories so that at a glance you can see which group they are from.

Allowed food groups

PROTEINS	CARBOHYDRATES	VEGETABLES
Lean chicken breast/mince (95% + lean)	Potato	Broccoli
Lean turkey breast/mince (95% + lean)	Sweet potato	Asparagus
Protein bars	Pumpkin	Lettuce
Low-fat cottage cheese	Rices White/Brown/Wild	Eggplant

PROTEINS	CARBOHYDRATES	VEGETABLES
BBQ chicken (skin removed)	Beans	Cauliflower
White fish	Peas	Squash
Squid	Carrots	Capsicum
Salmon	Pasta	Mushrooms
Tuna	Noodles (not 2-minute kind)	Spinach
Crab	Oatmeal	Brussels sprouts
Lobster	Barley	Cabbage
Prawns	Fruit	Celery
Lean turkey mince	Grainy bread	Cucumber
Lean red-meat 95%+	Tomato	Onion
Lean ham	Corn	Leek
Egg whites	Wholegrain cereals	Salad leaves
Fat-free yoghurt	Couscous	Asian greens
	Noodles/Mountain Bread wraps	Herbs

Note: If for any reason you are unable to be on or continue on a diet that encourages ketosis due to medical reasons, or you are obese or morbidly obese rather than overweight, then please look at adding 100 calories per meal from the centre column 'Carbohydrates'. This will ensure that you have boosted your calorie amounts for the day as well as added in a few sometimes-necessary carbohydrates. Check with your doctor or dietitian to see if this is necessary for you.

Recommended snacks

- ½ or ¼ of a protein bar (try mine, see *thenewme.com.au*)
- Celery or carrot sticks + 1 teaspoon of tahini (or avocado or mayonnaise instead)
- Strips of BBQ chicken (skin removed)
- Tossed salad
- Diet or low-fat yoghurt
- Diet or low-fat yoghurt sprinkled with 1 tablespoon LSA (ground linseed, sunflower and almond mix available from health food stores)
- Raw nuts (no more than 15)
- Natural peanut butter (ground nuts with no sugar or salt added) on celery sticks
- Light cottage cheese on celery or carrot
- Vegetable pieces (capsicum, celery, cucumber, broccoli florets, any crunchy vegetable of your choice) with avocado dip (¼ avocado mashed with 1 tablespoon low-fat cream cheese and cracked pepper)
- 3 tablespoons light cottage cheese mixed in with some cinnamon and Splenda (artificial sweetener) if you're after something sweet
- Glass of skim or low-fat milk
- 1 small piece of fruit such as an apple or a handful of berries or a handful of fruit and nut trail mix (when not restricting fruit)

7-Day menu plan shopping list

Please note that the research that has gone into the shopping list is based on items that are the lowest in certain things such as calories, salt, fat, carbohydrates and so on, not because of the price or brand name. You, can, of course, buy an alternative brand if you have a brand you prefer or can't find the ones listed – but remember that they may not be as low in salt, sugar, calories and fat. Make sure you read the labels to find the best product that suits your needs. You don't need all of the items listed to prepare the recipes, but they are good to stock in your pantry for creating your own Eat Smart Recipes. And to start afresh with a whole new pantry and kitchen of smart foods.

Note: The composition of the food products recommended can be subject to change.

Sauces and dressings

ABC sweet soy sauce (Kecap Manis)

All-natural tahini

Berri lemon squeeze

Berri lime squeeze

Chang's original Hoisin sauce

Chang's oyster sauce

Chang's pure sesame oil

Dolmio chunky vegetable pasta sauce

Fountain sweet chilli sauce

Fountain tomato sauce (no added salt)

Gravox light supreme salt reduced

Holbrooks Worcestershire sauce

Homebrand chunky pasta sauce

Homebrand white vinegar

Homebrand wholegrain mustard

Kikkoman soy sauce (43% less salt)

Leggo's pesto sauce

Leggo's tomato paste (no added salt)

Masterfoods chilli sauce

McIlhenny Co. Tabasco pepper sauce

Modena balsamic vinegar (Moro brand)

Poonsin fish sauce

Praise Caesar dressing 99% fat free

Praise creamy mayonnaise 97% fat free

Safeway brand lime coriander and chilli salad dressing

Herbs and spices

Continental chicken salt

Curry powder

Gourmet herb blend paste and herb squeeze tubes

Hoyt's minced garlic

Select brand dry herbs: parsley, basil, oregano, Italian herbs, ground ginger, coriander, paprika, cumin

Tuna (no oil)

Coles brand tuna flavours

Greenseas fat-free tuna flavours

Homebrand tuna in spring water

Nuts (make sure the ingredients list only the type of nut and no added oils)

Duck's pinenuts

Natural almonds

Natural cashew kernels

Raw macadamias

Cold foods

Bulla low fat cottage cheese 97% fat free

Nestlé Diet Yogurt

Pantalica smooth ricotta

Pauls 99.8% fat free natural yoghurt

Philadelphia extra light cream cheese

Tasmanian ultimate fetta reduced fat

Frozen foods

Birds Eye frozen steam-fresh vegetables

Birds Eye steam fish fillets in Thai coconut curry, lemon and parsley, garlic and spring onion, mild chilli

Pantry staples

bamboo skewers

breadcrumbs

cans of bamboo shoots

cans of diced tomatoes

cans of sliced water chestnuts

Kraft kalamata olives

LSA (ground linseed, sunflower and almond mix)

salt-reduced chicken stock

sesame seeds

(Less < Cal) Spray oil

Splenda low calorie sweetener

white wine

Drinks

Coke Zero

Diet Coke

Diet Sprite

Jarrah Hot Chocs in Chocolatte Frothy, Chocolatte Fudge, Chocolatte Caramel Dream, Chocolatte white chocolate

Pepsi Max

Waterford mineral water drink

Meat and seafood

barbecue chicken (skin removed)

chicken breast fillets

extra lean mince (beef)

lean chicken mince

turkey mince

low-fat shaved ham

salmon

tuna

white fish

prawns

squid

Vegetables

asparagus

avocado

baby spinach leaves

bean sprouts

bok choy

broccoli

broccolini

capsicum (red and green)

carrots (optional)

cauliflower

celery

chilli

cos lettuce

cucumber

eggplant

English spinach

garlic sprouts

green apples
  (for Thai salad)

iceberg lettuce

lettuce

mushrooms – button,
  field, oyster, shiitake

onions and red onions

rocket

snow peas

spring onions

squash

tomatoes (optional)

wombok (Chinese cabbage)

zucchini

Shopping list for Maintenance menu plan or Make-your-own menu plan or for those who can't or don't want to go into ketosis

barley

beans

bread, wholegrain

carrots

couscous

fruit (all types)

Mountain Bread wholewheat,
  rye (Light wraps)

oatmeal

noodles (not the 2-minute type)

pasta

peas

potatoes

pumpkin

rice: preferably brown,
  wild or basmati

spaghetti

sweet potato

tomatoes

Uncle Tobys Oats quick
  sachets

Wokka egg noodles

wonton wrappers/ gow gee
  pastry

Add your own Eat Smart foods:

Shopping is really important – probably the most important task of all – as it lays the foundations for your food and eating all week. Get this right, and you potentially have a great week. Get it wrong, and . . . gulp.

10 Grocery Shopping Tips

1. **Eat before you go.** Hunger is a distraction too! And can influence your choices of items or quantity.

2. **Go without the kids.** The fewer distractions you have, the better. I understand this may not be possible for everyone, but if you can try and take an hour out of your week to do this on your own, you'll have more time to reflect on your choices and explore new healthy choices. Soon you will automatically know what to grab, but for now give yourself the time.

3. **Make a grocery list throughout the week and add anything you might be running low on in your pantry, fridge or freezer.** Before you go shopping, take 15–20 minutes to plan your breakfasts, lunches and dinners for the week, adding any extra ingredients to your list.

4. **Make a budget and stick to it.** If you follow the first three steps you'll be saving money already. As you plan your meals, check supermarket ads for weekly specials, then stick to your list. Eating healthily can be economical when you portion differently and substitute processed or junk foods with vegies, salads and meat. Choose fresh, seasonal foods (fruit and vegetables in season are cheaper) over the latest kiddy-commercial junk food and pre-packaged snacks. Remember, you are shopping healthily *instead* of badly.

5. **Shop with a buddy.** Pair up with a similarly interested friend or family member. Learning together is more fun.

6. **Stick to the outside aisles at the supermarket.** The outside aisles contain the fresh food and more often than not most of the foods in the inside aisles of the supermarket are processed, packaged and not as healthy.

7. **Shop at specialty stores.** If you shop at a specialty store for specific items you will limit the number of sabotages and distractions you may face when shopping at a supermarket. Go to the butcher for meat, the poultry shop for chicken and the fishmonger for seafood as none of these stores have aisles of chocolates and lollies.

8. **Buy pre-cut, tinned or frozen vegetables.** Paying a little extra for pre-cut vegies will help guarantee that your family eats more of these healthy choices due to the convenience of being able to grab it without washing, peeling or cutting. And, remember that frozen or canned fruits and vegies are good for you, too. Just make sure to avoid added sugar (in fruits) and salt (in vegetables).

9. **Shop online.** It's an added cost for delivery but it definitely limits emotional shopping and prevents you (or the kids) from going crazy with the temptations at the checkouts.

10. **Shop in the right state of mind.** If you shop straight after a workout session, this will ensure you only shop healthily. (Can you imagine buying bad foods while still feeling pumped from your workout?) Use this method to have a fantastic shopping trolley every time.

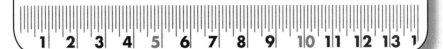

7-Day Menu Plan

Warning: This plan goes under the current recommendations put out by nutritional authorities. The current recommendation is for females not to go under 1200 calories, and males under 1800 calories when dieting. However, the suggested calorie allowance is to promote safe, but rapid weight loss, and is only to be done for a short period of time. Very Low Calorie Diets (VLCDs) go under 1000 calories, and are not to be done without medical supervision, but this calorie allowance is relatively low, rather than very low. It also takes into account any excess calories you might end up consuming from eating out, extra fats and slip-ups, so taking these things into account you probably won't end up eating the lowest calorie suggestion, anyhow. **YOU MUST check with your doctor or a dietitian before starting this plan to make sure it is right for you. If at, any time, you feel too hungry, simply increase the suggested serving sizes.**

Monday

Breakfast: Yoghurt and Nuts
Lunch: Prawn and Baby Spinach Salad
Dinner: San Choy Bau

Tuesday

Breakfast: Egg White Omelette
Lunch: Lemongrass Chicken and Vegetable Stir-Fry
Dinner: Salmon and Wasabi Yoghurt with English Spinach
  and Asparagus

Wednesday

Breakfast: Yoghurt and Prunes
Lunch: Warm Chicken Waldorf Salad
Dinner: Lettuce Spaghetti Bolognaise

Thursday

Breakfast: Flipped Omelette
Lunch: Teriyaki Calamari Skewers
Dinner: Chicken Meatloaf with Vegetables

Friday

Breakfast: Egg-white Omelette
Lunch: Thai Salad
Dinner: Pesto Fish with Cauliflower Mash

Saturday

Breakfast: Baked Eggs
Lunch: Caesar Salad
Dinner: Chicken Pizza with Mixed-leaf Salad

Sunday

Breakfast: Scrambled Eggs and Ham
Lunch: Chicken Skewers with Lemon Yoghurt
Dinner: Salmon Poached in White Wine with Salad

You can find the recipes for these meals in the 'Eat Smart Recipes' section on pages 197–215. Add 2–4 snacks from the snacks list on page 173. Change carbohydrates if necessary from the 'Allowed food groups' list on pages 171–2.

Make-Your-Own Menu Plan

If you find that the 7-Day Menu Plan doesn't fit in with your way of eating, simply adapt or create your own menu while still sticking to the suggested calorie limit. This will also prove important for those occasions when you can't cook at home and have to eat out or deal with special occasions.

Feel free to experiment with your diet: swap food items or complete recipes to make them more palatable or convenient to your lifestyle – this is what the Eat Smart Recipes on pages 197–215 are all about. There are stacks of recipe books out there listing the calorie content of meals that give you the opportunity to create your own smart way of eating.

Monday

Breakfast (around 200 calories)

Lunch (around 300 calories)

Dinner (around 300 calories)

Snacks (around 100 calories each)

Tuesday

Breakfast (around 200 calories)

Lunch (around 300 calories)

Dinner (around 300 calories)

Snacks (around 100 calories each)

Wednesday

Breakfast (around 200 calories)

Lunch (around 300 calories)

Dinner (around 300 calories)

Snacks (around 100 calories each)

Thursday

Breakfast (around 200 calories)

Lunch (around 300 calories)

Dinner (around 300 calories)

Snacks (around 100 calories each)

Friday

Breakfast (around 200 calories)

Lunch (around 300 calories)

Dinner (around 300 calories)

Snacks (around 100 calories each)

Saturday

Breakfast (around 200 calories)

Lunch (around 300 calories)

Dinner (around 300 calories)

Snacks (around 100 calories each)

Sunday

Breakfast (around 200 calories)

Lunch (around 300 calories)

Dinner (around 300 calories)

Snacks (around 100 calories each)

Maintenance Menu Plan

After you've reached your goal weight, you will need to work out a healthy food balance and reintroduce foods that you want to, such as carbohydrates, while still maintaining a healthy diet. But remember, this isn't a green light to return to your old way of eating. Instead:

- Reintroduce fruits, but make sure you're eating no more than two pieces of fruit a day.

- Reintroduce carbohydrates slowly, if you feel you need to.

- Choose wholegrain carbohydrates, such as wholemeal pasta, brown rice, and soy and linseed bread, which fill you up faster and keep you satisfied for longer.

- Have 2–3 times the amount of protein as carbohydrate to balance the sugars.

- Incorporate these fruits and carbohydrates into a calorie-controlled menu plan. You will get to the stage where you know what to eat automatically, without having to think about it, but just to make sure you have your skills down-pat before going it alone, design yourself a plan incorporating wholegrain carbohydrates, fruit, any of your favourite Eat Smart Recipes, as well as your own Eat Smart Recipes you have created by substituting ingredients to lower the fat, sugar, carbohydrate and calorie content.

Your Maintenance Calorie Quota

Once you're no longer trying to achieve a daily CD, a good rule for not gaining weight once you have reached your goal is to work on keeping your food intake at 300–500 calories below your TDEE (refer back to Calculating Calorie Deficits for your BMR and TDEE). To calculate your TDEE, simply multiply your BMR by your current physical activity levels (see page 159), which would now ideally be moderately–very active. (Aiming to eat just under your TDEE, allows for those inevitable times where you make a dietary slip-up or slack off with your exercise levels.)

Your Daily Maintenance Calorie Quota = (BMR x Current physical activity levels) -300–500 calories = _____ **calories**

Monday

Breakfast _____

Lunch _____

Dinner _____

Snacks _____

Tuesday

Breakfast _____

Lunch _____

Dinner _____

Snacks _____

Wednesday

Breakfast _____

Lunch _____

Dinner

Snacks

Thursday

Breakfast

Lunch

Dinner

Snacks

Friday

Breakfast

Lunch

Dinner

Snacks

Saturday

Breakfast

Lunch

Dinner

Snacks

Sunday

Breakfast

Lunch

Dinner

Snacks

Eating in the real world

One obstacle that we are almost certain to face until the end of time is the fact that we need to eat out – it may be a special occasion that we must attend, such as a work function, wedding or birthday party, or sometimes you just don't feel like cooking.

There is no problem with eating out, although if you do it too often it is sure to slow your weight loss progress. (It's helpful when starting on your weight loss journey to avoid eating out for at least a week so you don't get caught out making poor choices when you're trying to start a new way of eating; you want to set yourself off on the right foot.) But, with a few simple tips, you can make the most of eating out without blowing out in calories.

Tips for eating out

- Make sure that you either eat out at a healthy alternative café/restaurant or that you pull apart the menu to make sure that you are ordering and eating exactly what you want and nothing else.

- Order the meal how you want it cooked. You have the confidence to order your coffee exactly how you like it and you wouldn't think twice about sending it back because it wasn't made to your request, so why not do the same in a café/restaurant when ordering food?

- To make your special requests easier to ask for, imagine you are allergic to the items you cannot eat. You wouldn't think twice about asking for your food to be cooked without these items if they made you ill, so apply the same thinking to the items that would have ill effects on your weight loss.

- As a general rule, I would steer clear of particular restaurant types that make it very hard to order light; these restaurants would generally be Italian, Chinese and Indian. Eating at an Italian restaurant is okay if they have an extended menu including meat, seafood and chicken, which can be served with salad. If you must eat Chinese or Indian, order the leanest meal (no fried food or curries) and eat it without rice.
- Snack on salad or olives instead of bread while you wait for your meal.
- Ask for dressings to be put on the side and dip your fork, not your food, in the dressing, to get the taste without all the calories you would if you were to put the whole dressing on your salad.

The most important thing to be aware of during your dining experience is:

- You order what you want and you get what you order!

When reading the menu, don't get too caught up in what you see; there are many different things that you can order from what they already have on the menu or just by using the ingredients you see in different dishes and having them put it together as a meal for you.

Some questions to ask yourself and the wait staff after reading the menu are:

- Can the menu be modified to suit your dietary requirements?
- Do they have vegetables boiled or steamed? Make sure that the vegetables they have are not marinated or soaked in butter, honey or oil.

continued

- Can you replace any of the potato (or other carbs) on the plate with greens?
- Can you order your meal cooked with no oil ('I don't mind if it is slightly drier than the chef would like it to be')?
- Can you not get any drizzles of oil or garnishes of any kind?
- Can you get any jus, gravies, sauces in a small dish on the side?
- Do they do the meal in entrée size?

While any dish can be modified to suit your needs if you just think about it and ask for it there are a few little pointers that I would like to make you aware of:

- Calorie-wise, a plain salad will be your lightest calorie option.
- Seafood cooked fresh and light will always be your best calorie/protein option.
- Chicken is the second-best calorie meat option followed by red meats. When ordering chicken and meats it is important to ask for the cut to come with no skin on the chicken, and no fat on the meat. Ordering the meat to the size you want is also very important, and you will find that with each cut of meat available the relevant information is in your calorie books.

Always remember to make a trade off. You can't have an entrée and a main and a dessert and bread, pasta, rice or potatoes on the side; you have to choose <u>one</u> *treat! And, the smartest choice is one small nutritious meal, which you can savour slowly as you delight in the flavours of the meal, which will most likely be different from the meals you prepare at home – this is treat enough!*

Tips for special occasions, such as barbecues, dinner parties and festive gatherings

- Ask the host to remove some salad before they dress it.
- Skip the potato and pasta salads, or any salads with creamy dressings (or have just one tablespoon's worth to get the taste instead of the calories).
- Make sure there are meats available, other than fatty sausages and rissoles; try taking your own.
- Drink water instead of soft drinks.
- Eat before you go so you're not hungry at the party.

Cement in your mind that **you are not missing out.** All of the foods that you feel you have to miss out on while you're losing weight will still be there when you're done. You will not miss out on anything forever; it is just while you are losing the weight, the fewer things that tarnish your calorie deficit, the faster you will be rewarded for your efforts.

Tips for takeaway

While we now practise a new, smarter way of eating by being prepared when we go out, sometimes we are not

continued

going to be able to foresee running late, forgetting lunch, not having the ingredients at home or simply either not feeling like cooking or wanting to grab something on the way or while shopping.

I am not going to tell you that you absolutely cannot ever eat out again as that would just be ridiculous and unrealistic; so what I would like to do is make sure that you have a new outlook on what it is that you see and choose to eat if you are faced with the option of takeaway.

Here are some fast-food options or ideas that will make eating out or grabbing something on the run a little easier.

- Salad is the best choice, with no dressing (or dressing on the side) and any add-ins should be what you know you can eat, such as low-fat cheese, tuna, lean ham or grilled chicken, and should all be either small amounts cooked/prepared how you like them or not in there at all.

- Any sandwich store should be able to do you a salad in a bowl rather than on a roll or in a sandwich, including Subway. Sumo Salad bars are also a good choice, but just like with any salads you order, be careful of the dressings.

- Charcoal or barbecue chicken is the best option if you are looking for a substantial meal that's relatively healthy. (Of course, don't eat the skin and don't order chips or creamy pasta and potato salads that often accompany the chicken.) **Note:** The chicken must still resemble the actual bird; if it doesn't look like a piece of chicken, such as nuggets and chicken strips, then it's best to avoid because you can't be certain what else is in it.

- Kebabs are another reasonable way of grabbing something on the go. The way to order a kebab is on a plate, without the bread and to have the chicken as the meat filling (best fat choice). Get the meat trimmed while you watch to make sure it does not fall to the bottom of the tray, which is where the excess fat drips. All of the salads are dressing-free and if you want to you can still have a touch of tomato sauce or hoummos.

- If you don't have a choice other than a burger store, go for salads if they have them without the dressing, if a hamburger is your only option, eat only half the burger bun and take off greasy fillings such as cheese and bacon. (And, skip the fries, of course!)

- Thai food is generally a good choice for an Asian-style meal as is sashimi; both of these choices are quite light and flavoured with herbs and spices rather than oils, fats and creams – although be aware that curries are generally coconut milk or cream based, which have a high fat and calorie content.

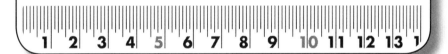

A typical example of how I would order some dishes

- Caesar Salad: No dressing (I don't order it on the side because I don't eat it anyway), no croutons, a runny egg (this ends up being my dressing) and go light on the bacon and cheese. Now this normally gets a laugh from the person taking the order but it is me who is eating it and this is how I enjoy my Caesar.

- Fish: White fish grilled, no oil and (generally) no flour, salad with no dressing (depending on the type of salad), no cheese (I don't eat many cheeses), no oils or drizzles on the plate (especially in expensive restaurants where they garnish more), and if I order vegetables no potato, corn, peas or beans and none of it to have any oils, butters or anything on the vegies, just boiled or preferably steamed.

- Things that I definitely do not even allow on my plate are things like chips, potato (mashed, baked, kipfler, baby chat, wedges, roasted, etc), gravies, sauces, dressings, bread.

- With desserts, sweets and treats, be aware of the calorie consequences and know that they are probably not going to be good for your journey. Remember that every obstacle you put in your way is another obstacle you have to work off.

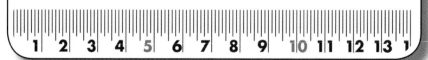

A calorie quiz for foods you might eat

Go through and answer the following questions:

1. Work out the calories for the following:

   A large Big Mac Meal with Coke _____

   A quarter of a barbecue chicken (skin off) and a garden salad with half a tomato _____

   3 Californian sushi rolls with tuna and soy sauce _____

   A regular chicken Caesar salad _____

   A chicken Caesar salad as Adro would order it

   _____

2. Write out three options the old you would choose from your local food court and work out the calories in them.

   - _____

   - _____

   - _____

   Now write some smarter alternatives to three old choices. These will be your new choices.

   - _____

   - _____

   - _____

3. When going out for dinner prepare for it by knowing roughly what you would like to eat and write down how you will be ordering it and approximately what the calories will be for that meal. Try previewing the menu where possible.

4. What are some of the key things to look for when you are going to be eating out.

Eat Smart Recipes

The Eat Smart Recipes are based on the philosophy that you can still enjoy old favourites by making some smart substitutions to reduce the fat, carbohydrate, sugar and calorie count. With simple substitutions of ingredients you can adapt any recipe to fit the Eat Smart principle: low calorie, low carb, low fat, high protein. Remember, this is about making smart choices within your current eating environment so start substituting your own ingredients and coming up with your own Eat Smart Recipes.

> *TIP* Tomatoes, carrots, apples and Mountain Bread wraps are optional ingredients. I recommend not eating these items (unless for personal preference or medical reasons you're allowing carbohydrates from the middle column of 'Allowed food groups' on page 171–2) for at least seven days, to give your body the best shot at eliminating all sugars, and reintroduce them later.

Breakfast

Baked Eggs

Portions	Ingredients
1	spray of oil (about a second)
3	egg whites, lightly beaten
1	slice of tomato (optional)
1 tbsp	low-fat cottage cheese
1	whole egg
1	spring onion, finely sliced

- Preheat oven to 200ºC.
- Put egg whites in a greased ramekin and gently place the tomato slice on top.

- Top with cottage cheese, whole egg and spring onions.
- Bake in oven for 15 minutes.

Tip: The tomato and spring onion can be substituted for any other ingredients such as mushroom, chicken, ham, capsicum, etc. Work the calories out accordingly.

- Serve in the ramekin when it is cooked (be careful as the ramekin will be hot).

Serves 1 @ 195 calories per serve

Egg White Omelette

Portions	Ingredients
1	spray of oil (about a second)
5	egg whites, lightly beaten
50 grams	cooked or barbecue chicken (no skin)
2	spring onions, finely sliced

For a choice of toppings:

¼	medium tomato, diced (optional)
1	capsicum cheek, sliced
1	medium mushroom, diced
	sprinkling of herbs, such as chives, chilli or garlic

- Spray omelette pan or frypan with oil and place over medium heat.
- Add your choice of toppings to the combined egg whites, chicken and spring onions, and place in the frypan for 10 minutes, turning sides as needed.

Tip: You can use any of the listed ingredients and work your calories out accordingly.

Serves 1 @ 190 calories per serve
(adjust calories according to chosen toppings)

Flipped Omelette

Portions	Ingredients
1	spray of oil (about a second)
5	egg whites (or 1 egg white and 1 whole egg)
1	spring onion, finely sliced
25 grams	low-fat shaved ham
1	medium mushroom, finely sliced

- Spray frypan with oil and place over medium heat.
- Pour egg whites into the pan and cook for 1 minute.
- Place filling ingredients over one half of the egg whites.
- With a spatula (egg flip) fold the empty side of the omelette over the half with the filling.
- Wait for the filling to heat through, then flip the omelette to brown the other side.

Tip: To practise flipping omelettes start by making smaller ones. Feel free to use any vegetable filling you like in the omelettes, just adjust the calories accordingly.

Serves 1 @ 177 calories per serve

Scrambled Eggs and Ham

Portions	Ingredients
1	spray of oil (about a second)
9	egg whites, lightly beaten
¼ cup	low-fat milk (optional)
1 tsp	dried oregano
4	slices low-fat ham (approx. 50 grams)
4	toothpicks

- Preheat oven to 200°C.
- Spray omelette pan or frypan with oil and place over medium heat.
- Mix the egg whites, milk and oregano, and pour into the frypan.
- With a whisk or fork scramble the eggs until all of the liquid has evaporated.
- Place the ham slices flat onto a chopping board and top with cooked egg mixture.
- Roll up the ham slices, and use a toothpick to hold their shape.
- Place in a baking dish and cook in the oven for 10 minutes.

Serves 2 @ 140 calories per serve

Alternative Breakfast Options

- Mix 200 grams of plain non-fat yoghurt with a handful of nuts (no more than 10–15) or 4–6 pitted prunes. Add a teaspoon of cinnamon and sweetener, if you like.
- Have one 200 gram flavoured diet or low-fat yoghurt.

Lunch and Dinner
Caesar Salad

Portions	Ingredients
2	slices Mountain Bread wraps (optional)
4	eggs (only whites will be used)
200 grams	barbecue chicken (skin removed), diced
200 grams	low-fat ham, diced
20	cos lettuce leaves, washed and sliced
4 tbsp	low-fat Caesar salad dressing

- Preheat oven to 200ºC.
- Cut the Mountain Bread into small triangular pieces and place on a baking tray. Bake for 3–5 minutes (keep an eye on it to ensure it doesn't burn).
- Place the eggs in a saucepan of boiling water. Boil for 5 minutes. Remove and cool.
- Place the chicken and ham into a frypan and heat through on medium heat, then remove.
- Divide the cos lettuce evenly among four plates.
- Peel the eggs and discard the yolks. Using the small holes on a cheese grater, grate the egg white, or slice, and sprinkle over the lettuce.
- Top with the chicken and ham, followed by the Mountain Bread crisps.
- Serve with a tablespoon of the dressing on the side to dip a fork into before adding salad. This allows you to taste the flavours of the salad, not just the dressing.

Tip: The bread crisps are not necessary; adjust your calories if you leave them out.

Serves 4 @ 220 calories per serve

Meatloaf with Vegetables

Portions	Ingredients
For the meatloaf	
500 grams	lean turkey or chicken breast mince
1	small carrot, diced (optional)
½	zucchini, diced
½	medium onion, diced
2	egg whites
1 tsp	crushed garlic
1 tsp	curry powder
1	spray of oil (about a second)
For the vegetables	
4	medium tomatoes (optional)
16	button mushrooms
1	spray of oil (about a second)

- Preheat oven to 200ºC.

For the meatloaf:

- Place all the meatloaf ingredients (except the oil spray) into a mixing bowl and mix together by hand until combined.
- Place the mixture into lightly greased loaf tin and place in the oven for 45 minutes.

For the vegetables:

- Place the tomatoes and mushrooms in a baking dish and lightly spray with oil.
- Place in the oven for the last 15 minutes of the meatloaf cooking time.
- To serve, cut the meatloaf into four slices and serve on a bed of cauliflower mash (see page 215) with a tomato and four mushrooms.

Tip: Tastes great with a drizzle of gravy but don't forget the extra 25 calories.

Serves 4 @ 265 calories per serve (including side of cauliflower mash)

Chicken Pizza

Portions	Ingredients
1	piece chicken breast (approx. 100 grams flattened out to 5 mm)
1	spray of oil (about a second)
1 tsp	pasta sauce or tomato paste
15 grams	low-fat tasty cheese, shredded
Toppings:	
1	medium mushroom, sliced
¼	medium tomato, diced
3	kalamata olives
20 grams	low-fat ham, sliced
1	capsicum cheek, diced
1	spring onion, finely chopped
5 grams	baby spinach, finely chopped

- Preheat oven to 190°C.
- Place the flattened chicken breast on a lightly greased oven tray.
- Spread the pasta sauce or tomato paste evenly over the chicken breast and top with your choice of toppings. (You can add other ingredients just remember to adjust the calories.)
- Finish off with a sprinkle of cheese and place in the oven for 15 minutes or until the cheese is slightly brown and melted.
- Serve with a mixed leaf salad.

Tip: To avoid making a mess, flatten the chicken breast with it inside a snaplock bag.

Serves 1 @ 245 calories per serve (including all listed toppings)

Chicken Skewers with Lemon Yoghurt

Portions	Ingredients
2 cups/500 grams	low-fat natural yoghurt
1 tsp	crushed garlic
2 tbsp	paprika
2 tbsp	cumin seeds
4 tbsp	lemon juice
2 tbsp	dried parsley
2 tbsp	dried oregano
	ground pepper to taste
3	sprays of oil (about 3 seconds)
1 kilogram	chicken breast fillets, cut into 2 cm cubes
18	bamboo skewers, soaked in warm water
200 grams	baby spinach

- Preheat grill to medium–high.
- Place the yoghurt, garlic, paprika, cumin seeds, lemon juice, parsley, oregano and pepper in a bowl and mix until combined. Place the mixture in two separate bowls. Use half of this mixture to coat the chicken pieces and chill the remainder to be used as a dipping sauce.
- Thread the chicken cubes evenly onto the skewers. Brush the chicken with some of the dipping sauce and cook for 5 minutes on each side.
- Serve skewers on top of a bed of baby spinach leaves.

Tip: Dipping sauce can be served in a bowl on the table with a spoon.

Serves 6 @ 258 calories per serve

Salmon Poached in White Wine with Vegetables and Mixed Salad

Portions	Ingredients
1	small carrot, julienned (optional)
4	broccoli florets
4	asparagus stalks, chopped
4	squash, halved
4	Atlantic salmon fillets (approx. 100 grams each)
1	sprig fresh rosemary, finely chopped
4 tsp	dried basil
1	pinch cracked black pepper
2	lemons, 1 cut into thin slices, 1 juiced
½ cup	white wine
4	slices of eggplant (1 cm thick), coated in pesto

- In a steamer, cook all the vegetables, except the eggplant, for 10–15 minutes.
- Place the fish in a shallow frypan over medium heat and sprinkle with the rosemary, basil and pepper.
- Cover the salmon with the lemon slices and carefully pour over the lemon juice and the wine.
- Cover the pan and poach for 5 minutes or until the fish changes colour.
- Fry the eggplant in a dry frypan over medium heat for 5 minutes.
- Serve the fish on top of the eggplant accompanied with the steamed vegetables, along with a mixed salad with no-oil dressing.

Tip: Salmon turns pale pink when cooked or will flake when tested with a fork.

Serves 4 @ 272 calories per serve

Lemongrass Chicken and Vegetable Stir-Fry

Portions	Ingredients
2	sprays of oil (about 2 seconds)
250 grams	chicken breast, diced
4 tbsp	sweet soy (kecap manis)
1	small carrot, julienned (optional)
¼	can water chestnuts, sliced
2	bok choys, roughly chopped
4	broccoli florets, roughly chopped
½	medium red onion, finely sliced
1 tsp	dried coriander
1 tbsp	chopped lemongrass
	water as needed

- Spray a heated wok with oil and add the chicken along with half of the quantity of soy sauce until just cooked. Remove from the wok and set aside in a warm place.
- Cook the vegetables, except for the bok choy, in the wok using the remaining sauce.
- When all the vegetables are tender, add bok choy, coriander and lemongrass and return the chicken to the wok.
- If necessary, add splashes of water while cooking to prevent the food from sticking, burning or drying out.
- Add noodles, such as soba noodles, when allowing carbohydrates (adjust calories accordingly).

Tip: Add bean shoots in the last few minutes to give a noodle texture when not using real noodles.

Serves 2 @ 245 calories per serve

Lettuce Spaghetti Bolognaise

Portions	Ingredients
1.2 kilograms	lean turkey or chicken breast mince
10	garlic shoots, finely diced or
1	tbsp crushed garlic
2 tbsp	dried oregano
2 tbsp	dried basil
2 tbsp	parsley, chopped
2 tbsp	Italian herbs
2	cans diced tomatoes (optional)
2	jars pasta sauce (optional)
2	iceberg lettuces, finely shredded
4	medium zucchini, finely diced
1	medium onion, finely diced
1	eggplant, finely diced
1	red capsicum, finely diced
4	mushrooms, finely diced
50 grams	baby spinach, finely diced
1	broccoli, finely diced

- Place the mince, garlic and all the herbs into a large frypan or saucepan and cook until the mince turns white (don't brown).
- Add the tomatoes and pasta sauce (replace with 2 cups of chicken stock if eliminating tomatoes) and stir through. Then add the remaining vegetables, except the lettuce and stir.
- Add in a tomato can measure of water and cook on medium–high for 30-40 minutes, stirring frequently.
- Serve 2 scoops of bolognaise over a bed of shredded lettuce. Add a dollop of low-fat ricotta (optional – adds 25 calories).

Serves 10 @ 295 calories per serve

Pesto Fish

Portions	Ingredients
3	zucchini, thinly sliced
16	cherry tomatoes (optional)
½	medium red onion, thinly sliced
¼ cup	fresh parsley, chopped
	pepper to taste
4	white fish fillets
¼ cup	pesto

- Preheat grill.
- Place the zucchini, tomatoes, onion and parsley on a lightly greased baking tray.
- Cook under the hot grill for approximately 8 minutes or until the zucchini is tender and the tomatoes begin to split. Season with pepper and cover to keep warm.
- Place the fish on a lightly greased oven tray and divide the pesto evenly over the top of the fish.
- Cook under the hot grill for approximately 8 minutes or until the fish is cooked through.
- Serve the fish with the grilled vegetables and a side of cauliflower mash (see page 215)

Tip: The fish will flake when tested with a fork when cooked.

Serves 4 @ 258 calories per serve (including side of cauliflower mash)

Prawn and Baby Spinach Salad

Portions	Ingredients
6–8	medium fresh prawns
1 tsp	crushed garlic
100 grams	baby spinach leaves
¼	large avocado, diced
½	medium red onion, sliced thinly
6	olives in brine
2 tbsp	balsamic vinegar

- Peel, de-vein and butterfly the prawns and cook in a non-stick hot pan with the crushed garlic.
- Rinse and dry the baby spinach and place on a plate.
- Layer the avocado, onion, olives and prawns on top of the spinach and drizzle with balsamic vinegar.

Serves 1 @ 285 calories per serve

Salmon and Wasabi Yoghurt

Portions	Ingredients
2	sprays of oil (about 2 seconds)
4	Atlantic salmon fillets (approx. 100 grams each)
2 tbsp	reduced-salt soy sauce
1 tsp	sesame oil

For the wasabi yoghurt:

Portions	Ingredients
1 cup	low-fat natural yoghurt
1 tsp	wasabi paste
1 tsp	grated ginger
½	lemon or lime, juiced
1 bunch	English spinach (approx. 300 grams)
12	asparagus spears

- Preheat oven to 100ºC.
- Lightly spray a baking dish with oil. Place the salmon in a single layer in the baking dish.
- Combine the soy sauce with the sesame oil and brush over the fillets.
- Bake for 20 minutes or until the salmon is cooked through.

For the wasabi yoghurt:

- Place the yoghurt, wasabi paste, ginger and lemon/lime juice in a bowl and mix to combine. Refrigerate until ready to serve.
- Steam or blanch the spinach until it is just wilted.
- Steam asparagus spears.
- Serve the spinach onto four plates, top with the salmon and asparagus, and accompany with wasabi yoghurt.

Serves 4 @ 262 calories per serve

San Choy Bau

Portions	Ingredients
600 grams	chicken breast mince
½	can water chestnuts, finely diced
½	can bamboo shoots, finely diced
2	mushrooms, finely diced
6	spring onions, finely chopped
1 tsp	crushed garlic
1 pinch	dried coriander
2 tbsp	rice wine vinegar
2 tbsp	sweet soy sauce (kecap manis)
2 tbsp	Hoisin sauce
1	chilli, deseeded and diced
½ cup	bean sprouts, chopped

| 4–8 | baby cos lettuce or iceberg lettuce leaves |
| 4 tbsp | fresh coriander leaves |

- Cook the chicken mince in a frypan or wok until cooked right through (when cooked it should be white).
- Add the water chestnuts, bamboo shoots, mushrooms, spring onions and garlic. Stir through the mince until cooked.
- Add the dried coriander, vinegar, soy and Hoisin sauces and cook for a further 2 minutes.
- Take the mixture off the heat and stir through the chilli and bean sprouts.
- Scoop the mixture from the wok or pan into washed lettuce cups. Top with fresh coriander and serve.

Serves 4 @ 211 calories per serve

Teriyaki Calamari Skewers

Portions	Ingredients
10	bamboo skewers, soaked in warm water
2	calamari tubes, cleaned and cut into 1 cm thick rings (500 grams makes approx. 20 rings), soaked in milk
200 grams	baby spinach leaves
For teriyaki sauce:	
3	spring onions, finely sliced
1 tsp	ginger, grated
¼ cup	red wine vinegar
2 tbsp	reduced-salt soy sauce
1 tbsp	sweet soy sauce (kecap manis)
2 tbsp	lemon or lime juice
1 tsp	sesame oil

- Soak the calamari in milk for as long as possible before using.
- Preheat grill to high.
- Slice calamari rings at one end to make strips, thread onto skewers in an 's' shape concertina and set back in milk until needed. (Use two rings per skewer or one ring per skewer to make a larger quantity for guests.)
- Remove calamari skewers from milk and drain. Place skewers under grill for 1 minute or until cooked.
- Serve hot on a bed of spinach leaves and drizzle with teriyaki sauce.

For the teriyaki sauce:

- Place the spring onions, ginger, vinegar, soy sauce, kecap manis and 1 tbsp of the juice in a small saucepan over medium heat. Heat, then stir in the sesame oil and remaining juice.

Tip: Soaking the calamari in milk prevents it from toughening; don't cook it for too long or it will become chewy.

Serves 2 @ 304 calories per serve

Thai Salad

Portions	Ingredients
For the salad:	
1	large wombok (Chinese cabbage), finely shredded
8	celery sticks, finely sliced
4	spring onions, finely sliced
4	large green apples, diced (optional)
For the dressing:	
½ cup	white vinegar
¼ cup	Splenda (or other liquid sweetener)
2 cups	sweet soy sauce (kecap manis)

| ¼ cup | reduced-salt soy sauce |
| ¾ cup | hot water |

For the salad:

- Mix all the ingredients together in a large salad bowl.

For the dressing:

- Into a 1 litre bottle, pour vinegar, Splenda (or other liquid sweetener), sweet soy and soy sauces. Put on the lid and shake well.
- Remove the lid and add near-boiling water to thin dressing.
- Serve with grilled chicken strips, barbecue chicken or lean meat or fish and 30 ml of dressing per serve. (Refrigerate remaining dressing for later use.)

Serves 4 @ 185 calories per serve
(adjust calories accordingly with added meat or fish)

Warm Chicken Waldorf Salad

Portions	Ingredients
For the salad:	
1	whole cooked or barbecue chicken, (skin removed) roughly chopped
4	medium green apples, cut into 2 cm chunks
100 grams	walnuts
12	large celery sticks, sliced
3	baby cos lettuce, sliced
200 grams	baby spinach
	spray of oil (about a second)
For the dressing:	
¼ cup	light sour cream
¼ cup	light mayonnaise
	pepper to taste

- Place a frypan over medium heat and add the chicken, apples and walnuts; heat through but don't overcook.

For the dressing:

- Mix the sour cream, mayonnaise and pepper until combined and smooth.
- Place all the ingredients in a large salad bowl and mix until combined, making sure to lightly coat all the ingredients with the dressing.

Tip: Add water to thin the dressing if necessary.

Serves 6 @ 318 calories per serve

Fast Lunch and Dinner Options

- Tuna mixed in with salad and balsamic vinegar and fat-free mayonnaise.
- 100–150 grams of chicken or very lean meat, grilled, barbecued, dry-fried in a non-stick frypan or baked with garlic or mixed spices (such as oregano, parsley, rosemary, thyme, sage) plus unlimited salad with a no-oil dressing.
- Any type of fish with lemongrass, chilli, coriander, dill, paprika, cumin or parsley, and lemon wrapped in foil plus steamed vegetables with 1 teaspoon of tahini.
- Cook vegetables, onion and herbs in water and low-salt chicken stock to make a soup.
- Make a ham and salad roll, by wrapping lean ham and salad ingredients in a piece of lettuce instead of bread.

Side Dishes

Cauliflower Mash

Portions	Ingredients
½	cauliflower (approx. 500 grams), chopped
2 tbsp	Philadelphia cream cheese 5% fat
1 tsp	crushed garlic
	pepper to taste

- Place the cauliflower in a pot of boiling water and allow to cook until soft.
- Drain well and place into a food processor or blender. Add the cream cheese and garlic and blend until smooth.
- This is a fantastic side dish that goes amazingly with most meals.

Tip: Add a little water, not too much, if necessary to aid blending; add parsley for a splash of colour.

Serves 4 @ 52 calories per serve

Fast Side Dish Options

- To make a mixed-leaf salad, mix greens with a dressing made of 1 teaspoon of seeded or Dijon mustard mixed with lemon juice or vinegar.
- Make any salad combination from your allowed vegetables tossed with no-oil dressing.
- Bake (cut the vegetables into chunks) or grill (cut the vegetables into thin slices) any vegetables from your allowed vegetables with a spray of oil; add herbs or chilli if you desire.
- Steam or stir-fry (using a non-stick frypan and a bit of water or oil spray) allowed vegetables. Steaming and stir-frying rather than boiling is best for retaining nutrients.

MOVE MORE PROGRAM

You are in total control of your success.

The Move More Program, like the Eat Smart Diet, is simple and flexible so that you can adjust it when you need to in order to fit your level of training and develop at your own pace. This will help you build a load of skills such as managing your training to suit your current fitness level, and when you're ready to progress, you have control over when to up the ante on your routine as well as how much of an increase in activity you are comfortable with. This gives you the satisfaction of knowing that you are in total control of your success.

The Move More Program is based on walking, running and resistance exercises using your own body weight because these ways of working out are simple, free and accessible to everyone. You will have no excuses like 'I can't afford a gym membership or exercise equipment' to not start straightaway. The program consists of a Walk Plan and a Circuit Plan.

- The Walk Plan walks you through a series of steps to increase your walking fitness by first going further, then going faster, by doing interval training. There are also guidelines to build up to running.

- The Circuit Plan is divided into two categories: upper body and lower body, and you alternate between an exercise for each category. The reason for this is that by alternating between upper and lower body exercises your heart has to work harder to move the blood to the muscles being worked, because they are at opposite ends of the body, this means you get your heart rate higher, which means you burn more calories. The plan is further divided into upper body, abdominal, lower body and full body because you'll have to switch between exercises on the ground and standing up – getting up and down repeatedly, raises your heart rate too.

Program guidelines

What?

You don't need to go to a gym to work out because there are more than enough things around in your everyday community that can be used for free, things like streets, parks, walking tracks, beaches and so on.

I am not discouraging the use of a gym by any means. I'm just well aware of the fact that lots of people wouldn't feel comfortable walking into a gym when they know they will have to face a gym full of thin and already fit people. If you are already a member of a gym you will be able to access the guidance of the fitness staff.

If you prefer, you can simply switch the program to fit cycling using cardio equipment in a gym, boxing or swimming and an alternate resistance program such as a circuit class at the gym or a weights program guided by a personal trainer or gym staff. It's not so much 'what you do', but 'how much you do'.

How much?

I recommend doing **at least an hour of exercise a day, seven days a week**. And, if you're really eager, then aim to do an hour, twice a day. **Note:** This is in addition to being more active by doing everyday things such as cleaning the house and taking the stairs. Your hour can also be divided up into half an hour in the morning and half an hour at night, or whatever kind of combination works for you in order to make this happen.

If this daily amount doesn't seem feasible, choose one day like a Saturday or Sunday where you can do a 2-hour session – before you baulk at this, just think a simple bike ride with your family for an hour followed by a walk or Frisbee throwing on the beach and you've easily made up your quota. Whatever way you make up your quota I recommend you aim for **a total of at least 7 hours of exercise a week**.

Remember, the more you do, the more you burn, and the more you benefit!

How hard?

A simple way to measure your exercise intensity is to use the Talk Test.

- **Low intensity** = You can talk easily, without taking a big breath in between sentences.

- **Moderate intensity** = You can still maintain a breathy conversation.

- **High intensity** = You're struggling to get a sentence out without taking a big full breath.

If you want to be more advanced and like using gadgets, a heart rate monitor is a great way to gauge intensity. Basically your Working Heart Rate Range (WHRR) needs to be around 60 and 80 per cent of your Maximum Heart Rate (MHR). A heart rate monitor will work this out for you. If you don't have one and you're interested in working it out manually, here's how to do it:

- To work out your MHR, simply subtract your age from 220 for females or 226 for males.

- Your WHRR is 60–80 per cent of this figure. So for me I was 26 during my time on *The Biggest Loser,* and my equation looked like this:

226–26 = 200
60–80% = (200 x 0.6)–(200 x 0.8)
WHRR = 120–160 bpm (beats per minute)

Once you know your WHRR you may want to stop periodically during your workout to check your heart rate and make sure you're in the zone. To take your pulse, place two fingers on the underside of your wrist or the side of your neck, count the number of beats you feel in 15 seconds, multiply this number by four and you get an estimation of the amount of beats per minute (bpm). It doesn't matter if you're a little over the 80 per cent mark, just as long as you're not within 10 per cent of your MHR. For high-intensity exercise your range will probably be 75–85 per cent and for lower intensity workouts your range will probably be 65–75 per cent.

When do I have to increase the intensity?

You will find that as time goes by you will have to increase the intensity of your walking, due to the fact that it will get too easy as you become fitter and you will burn less calories than you once used to doing the same activity, which means both your fitness and weight loss will slow up as a consequence. The same will be true for your circuits: the exercise you once struggled with will get easier as you get stronger so you will have to make the exercise harder or do more repetitions.

You will get to the stage when you're enjoying if not the exercise then at least the results the exercise is giving you, and this should spur you on to push yourself further. (Aiming to increase your workout every couple of weeks is a good guide.)

What is interval training?

Interval training is simply alternating between intervals of time where you push yourself to work harder followed by a recovery period where you slow down and get ready for the next interval. This is the type of training that I was murdered with, but I owe my fast improvements in fitness to my trainers.

Doing interval training is such a great training tool as it gets your body to start doing what is called 'Active Recovery'.

Active Recovery is when you have a spike in your heart rate, like say when you run a little, and then instead of stopping to rest and recover and get your heart rate and breathing under control you simply slow down to recover until you're ready to go again – you recover while you're still being active, hence the name. (I couldn't believe that I could rest without stopping either, but it's true!)

This way of training is so effective that many university studies have found that it really is the fastest and most effective method for losing the most fat and increasing fitness. This way of working out will seriously increase your fitness, which will make any other activities you end up doing easier, and you will notice the difference in no time at all.

How do I warm up and cool down?

Warming up and cooling down helps you prevent injuries and recover for tomorrow's sessions. If you're training outdoors, warm up with an introductory walk, starting at a slightly-faster-than-window-shopping pace, then speed it up over the time of your warm up until you're pretty much ready to walk fast or run – usually about 10 minutes. If you're indoors, increase the pace gradually in the same way using cardio equipment such as a treadmill or stationary bike. 'Warming into' your workout this way, prepares your muscles for the workout ahead. Finish your workout with the stretching routine provided later in the chapter (pages 236–9).

Training Plans

The training plans, at a glance:

- Do at least 7 hours of exercise a week.
- Do 6 hours a week of walking and/or running (or another type of cardio) from the Walking Plan.
- Do 2 x 30-minute circuit sessions from the Circuit Plan.
- Do 5–10 minutes of stretching after your workouts, using the allocated stretches.
- Break your workouts into smaller chunks of time if necessary.
- If you want to accelerate weight loss, increase to 2 hours a day, i.e. 14 hours a week.
- Aim to keep your heart rate above 140 bpm **(check with your doctor that this heart rate is safe for you)**, or at a minimum of a moderate intensity using the Talk Test, for the bulk of your workouts.
- Begin with what you can manage and build up gradually.
- When doing the exercises, start with the easiest version, and progress to the harder version when you're able and ready.
- Once a workout becomes easy you must increase the intensity by following the 'Stepping It Up' guidelines.

WARNING: If you're obese or morbidly obese, have high blood pressure, a chronic illness or are completely inactive, you must see a doctor or qualified personal trainer/exercise physiologist before commencing any of these training plans.

Walking Plan

- Start with what you can, but walking for at least 30 minutes a day is a good place to begin.

- Set yourself a course that you would like to walk each day. Choose a distance that you're comfortable with and then start walking it. Time how long it takes you. To improve your fitness and continue to lose weight, step it up a notch by outdoing the previous time each week.

- When you get your time down to about half of what it was when you first started it's time to step it up again by increasing the distance so it takes you back up to the original time. This is a really easy way of managing your increase in activity because before you know it the course you were doing is so easy that you wonder how you ever struggled with it – it may not happen in the first few days but definitely in a month or so and the more you follow this pattern the faster you will find yourself making progress. This noticeable progress gives you encouragement.

- Another option is to set a time limit of at least 30 minutes and try to walk further each week in the same amount of time. This is a little harder if you are walking around a block, and the end is where you started. Plan ways of how you can go further. For example, if you head out and turn left to walk around the block – front door to front door – walk about halfway, turn around and complete the full block ending back at your front door, this way you have actually walked it one-and-a-half times. Then you can walk a little further than halfway (when you're ready) before turning around at three-quarters and so on.

- Keep increasing the distance and speed until you are walking for 60 minutes.

- Walk fast enough. If you find it hard to talk then generally speaking you are going at a reasonable enough pace; if you have your heart rate monitor (HRM) on then you want to go somewhere above 140 bpm (now this, of course, depends on your age and weight so please check with your doctor).

Stepping It Up

- Once you've progressed your walking speed and distance, and you're walking for 60 minutes a day, you will need to up the ante another way (otherwise you'll end up having to walk all day or to the moon in order to keep progressing!). You can do this by introducing interval training to all or a few of your walks (if you choose to keep walking for 60 minutes for some of your walks, without interval training, increase the challenge by aiming to walk for longer or wearing a weighted vest).

- Find a hilly route to walk because the intervals are in-built: you have to work harder to climb the hill and then you recover as you go downhill, followed by walking on flat ground so you've recovered before you have to head up the next hill.

- Find some stairs: try a train station, school or sporting ground with stairs in the grandstand. Walk up the set of stairs slowly and walk back down even slower. Do this for 5–10 minutes at your own pace. Note how many flights of stairs you make and then each week try to increase the number of steps or flights you're able to climb in 5–10 minutes, meaning you'll have to go faster. Once you're moving at a reasonably fast pace, aim to do it for a longer time. You could use the same system to go up and down a hill.

- If you're walking on a street lined with telegraph poles, you might alternate between walking fast, power walking or even a light jog if you're up to it, between two poles (providing they're no more than 50 metres apart) and then walking slowly to recover for the next three poles. If this is too tough, do a 5:1 ratio (walk fast in between one set of poles, slowly for five poles and so on; five easy intervals: one hard interval) or just do fast walks randomly as you feel ready for each one. As you get fitter, you can reduce the rest intervals until you're up to a 1:1 ratio.

- Once you've progressed to a 1:1 ratio you can introduce some running. Simply run for as long as you can, walk to recover, run for as long as you can, walk to recover and so on – each week aiming to bridge the gap between time spent running and walking until you're able to run 5 minutes, then 10, then 20, then 30 minutes without stopping.

- Once you can run for 30 minutes without stopping, introduce the same interval training methods again, only this time you will be doing the intervals with running instead of walking.

Circuit Plan

- Incorporate at least two circuits a week of 30 minutes on top of your cardio.

- Simply choose an exercise from each category – upper body, abdominal, lower body and full body – and do each exercise 10–20 times or for 1 minute with little to no rest in between.

- Repeat this circuit at least three times, taking a few minutes to rest or walk in between each set.

- As you get fitter, take less rest and complete more sets of the circuit, until you're able to complete six circuits, with a 30–60-second breather in between each set.

- At first, choose exercises that you're able to do and prefer to do (I say 'prefer' because I don't expect you to ever like exercises like push-ups or squats). Before long you will find that the exercises you're doing have become a lot easier, so it is then that you can challenge yourself by trying new exercises.

- You can be as creative with putting your own circuit together as you like. You may just stick to repeating circuits of the same exercises for each category or you may do different exercises for each category with each set you do. Remember this is your opportunity to create a workout that suits you.

Stepping It Up

- Aim to complete more repetitions in 1 minute.
- Try a harder version of the exercise.
- Choose different exercises that challenge you more.
- Add more resistance to each exercise.

- Do more sets until the circuit takes you 45 minutes to complete.
- Vary the circuit and increase the cardio challenge by getting some plastic cones or bowls and writing the exercises on the bowls. Put them on the ground, 15–20 good paces apart and run between each marker, stopping to do the exercise at each one. The configuration can be anything you want, such as a clock shape, run to the centre and out again, using trees in the park and running, put the bowls in a straight line or run half of them parallel so it's like a shuttle run between them as you make your way down the line of exercises.

Maintenance Exercise Plan

- You must continue doing at least 30–60 minutes of activity each and every single day, for the rest of your life.
- The key is to find exercises that you enjoy so that you're likely to stick to it for life.
- Have faith; you will begin to enjoy exercise – I did.

Exercises and stretches

Note: When doing resistance exercises, breathe out on the exertion phase (the one where you have to apply the effort, such as pushing yourself up out of a push-up), and breathe in on the easy or preparation phase (such as lowering your chest down to prepare for a push-up). Never hold your breath.

Upper Body

Push-ups: Place your hands and toes on the ground, hands just wider than shoulder width apart. Tuck your backside under so your torso makes a straight line with the ground. Bend your elbows outwards as you lower your chest towards the ground. Without hunching your shoulders, push back up by straightening the elbows and repeat.

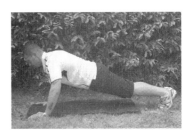
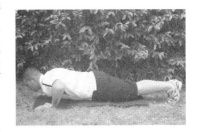

Make it easier

- Stand up and place your hands on a wall (easiest) or something a little lower like the back of a park bench or kitchen bench.
- Place knees on the ground.

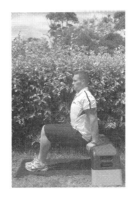

Bench dips: Sit on the edge of a bench with palms on the bench, fingers curled over the edge and knees bent, feet flat. Lift your backside off the bench, holding your weight through your hands. Keep shoulders drawn down, bend elbows pointing backwards to lower your body, push back up and repeat. Don't let your shoulders drift up towards your ears.

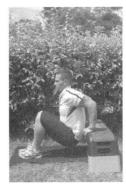

Make it harder

Place feet out in front, legs straight.

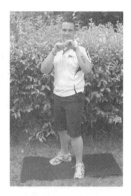

Air boxing: Keep elbows slightly bent, hands held in loose fists and punch the air with short, sharp jabs – vary the punching position between high punches and chest height. Make it harder: punch faster and harder.

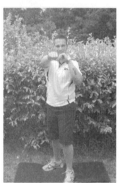

Abdominal and Core

Crunches: Lie on your back, knees bent and feet flat, and hands on your thighs. Bring your chest towards your knees, as far as you can go. Lower while maintaining stomach tension, and repeat.

Variations

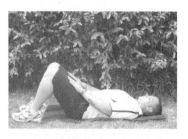

Side crunches: Lie on your side with knees bent. Complete crunches with hands underneath your neck, elbows out. Repeat for the other side.

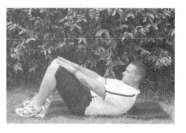

Reverse crunches: From the basic crunch position, place your hands by your sides on the ground. Squeeze into the lower part of your abdominals to lift your backside off the ground, lower and repeat.

Plank (Hover): Prop yourself up on your toes and forearms so your whole body makes a straight line, parallel to the ground. Squeeze your stomach muscles and hold, without holding your breath. Do not let your stomach sag or your backside drift up into the air.

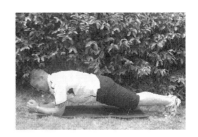

Make it easier

Drop your knees onto the ground so your torso is diagonal to the ground (place a rolled towel or cushion under your knees if you are uncomfortable).

Alternate arms and legs: Lie on your front, legs together and arms outstretched directly in front of you. Lift up your opposite arm and leg at the same time. Lower and lift the opposite arm and leg. Repeat, alternating sides. Keep your head in line with your spine.

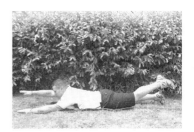

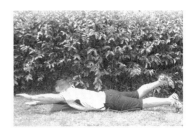

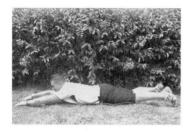

Superman: Lie on your front with arms stretched out in front – as if you were flying like Superman! Lift up your upper body and arms at the same time as your feet. Lower and repeat.

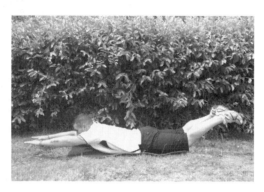

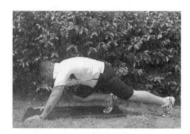

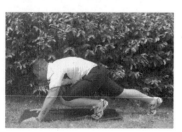

Lower Body

Mountain climbers: Place your hands on the ground or on a small step, shoulder width apart, toes on ground. Drive one knee forward up under your chest, push it back straight as you drive the other knee forward and so on.

Squats: Stand with feet just wider than hip-width apart. Bend your knees and lower your backside down and out as if you were about to sit back on a chair. Do not bend your knees forward over your toes; think 'sit into the squat'. Push back up and repeat.

Make it harder

- Piggyback someone.

- Hold the squat at the bottom and pulse up and down for 10–30 seconds.

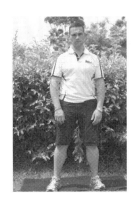
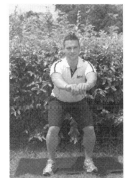

Step-ups: Step up onto a step, step back down and repeat. Do the same amount of step-ups leading with each leg. Be sure to place your whole foot on the step.

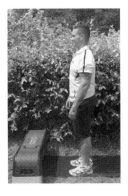
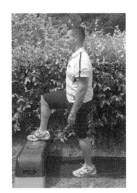
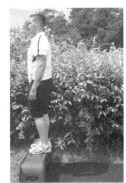

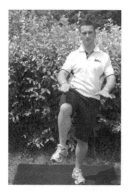

Knee lifts (High knees): Stand tall, lift one knee up to hip height, then the other and repeat.

Make it harder

Do this while running on the spot.

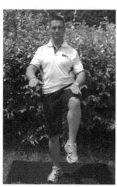

Side steps: Step out to the side, tapping your toes together. Step back to the other side and repeat.

Make it harder

- Add a clap with your hands as you tap your toes together.

- Keep your ankles together, as if you had rope tied around them, and take little jumps from side to side.

- Jump over a small object like a pair of rolled up socks or a shoe.

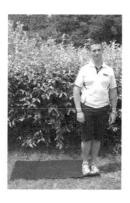
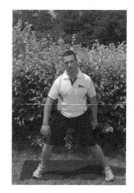

Scissor kicks: With a little jump, kick one foot forward and the other back. With another little jump, swap sides and repeat. Keep your legs as straight as possible.

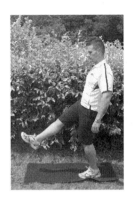

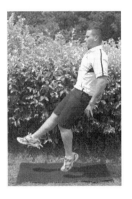

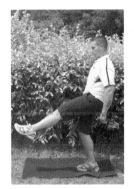

Skate: Lean forward, step from side to side, taking wide steps and swinging your arms outstretched, like you would if you were rollerblading or ice skating.

Make it harder

- Do a little jump to each side.
- Tap your heel behind you with your opposite hand.

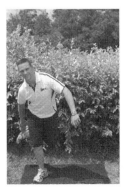
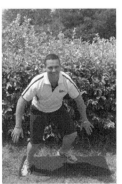
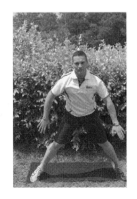

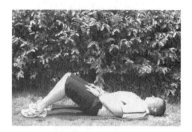

Full Body

Lie downs: Sit down, lie down (front or back) and get up. If you're overweight, getting up and off the ground is a good exercise in itself.

Make it harder

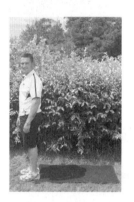

Do burpies: Squat down, place your hands on the ground out in front of you, jump your legs back, finishing up on your toes. Jump your knees back into your chest, bringing your toes back up towards your hands. Stand up and repeat again.

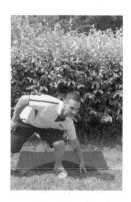

Shuttle sprints: Set two markers or shoes up, over about 10 metres, and run between them as fast as you can.

Make it harder

Bend down and touch the ground at each marker.

Star jumps: Jump, spreading your arms and legs out. Jump to bring your feet back together and arms by your sides, and repeat.

Make it easier

Just use your legs, keeping hands on hips.

Make it harder

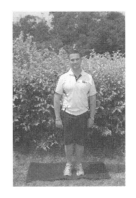

- Jump higher and take your arms up higher.
- Do them faster.

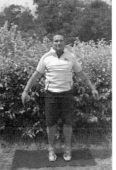

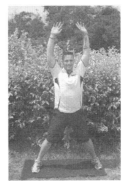

Air skipping: Do the action of skipping, but without a rope – vary the skipping style between single jumps, double jumps, shifting your weight from side to side and running skips.

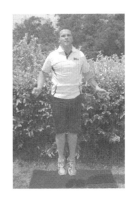

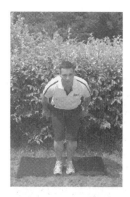

Vertical jumps: Bend down, jump up as high as you can.

Make it harder

Reach your hands up high as you jump.

Make it easier

Do a few jumps, and recover by repeating the same action without letting your feet lift off the ground.

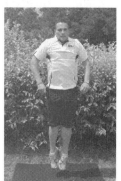

Stretches

Note: Hold stretches for 10–30 seconds. Relax and breathe while holding a stretch. You should feel the stretch without discomfort.

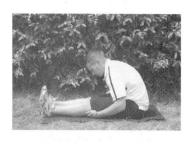

Rear-leg stretch: Sit on the ground with legs straight, toes pointing up. Bend from your hips, bringing head as far down as possible and hold.

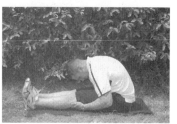

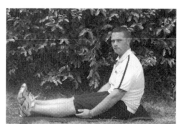

Quad stretch: Grab one foot, bend your knees slightly and bring your foot as close to your backside as possible, keeping knees in line, until you feel the stretch down the front of your thigh. You may need to hold on to something with the other hand for balance. Then, for an extra stretch into the front of your hip, without bending your torso forward pull your knee behind the line of the other knee. Repeat for the opposite side.

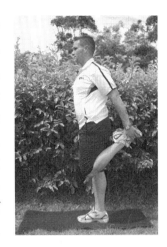

Glute stretch: Stand on one leg, with your opposite foot placed on the knee. Bend the knee on the standing leg and lean forward until you feel a stretch in your hip and outer backside on the side of the elevated leg. Use your elbow to push your knee towards the ground to intensify the stretch. Hold onto something if you need extra balance. Sit on a chair to make it easier. Repeat on the other side.

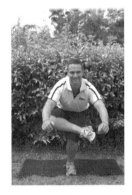

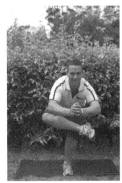

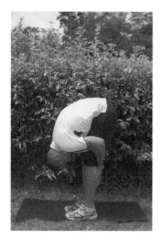

Hugging stretch: Stand straight with knees slightly bent, bend forward, grabbing the back of your legs, gently pulling your head towards your knees, until you feel the stretch down your back.

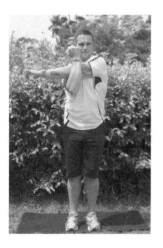

Shoulder and arm stretch: Place one arm across your chest, use the opposite arm to grab the elbow on the outstretched arm, pulling your elbow in towards your chest. Repeat using opposite arm.

Chest stretch: Cup fingers together behind your back. Lift your arms up without leaning forward and push your chest out until you feel your chest stretch.

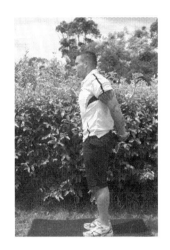

Neck stretch: Gently tilt your head to the right side, place your right hand onto your left ear and gently pull your head down towards your right shoulder. Release pressure off your neck before letting go with your hand and switching sides.

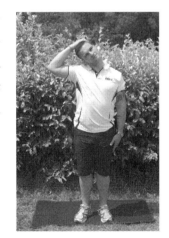

WORKSHOP: Circuit Template

Select one exercise from each category in the previous exercises to design your own circuit.

Set 1

Upper Body exercise:

Abdominal exercise:

Lower Body exercise:

Full Body exercise:

Set 2

Upper Body exercise:

Abdominal exercise:

Lower Body exercise:

Full Body exercise:

Set 3

Upper Body exercise:

Abdominal exercise:

Lower Body exercise:

Full Body exercise:

Set 4

Upper Body exercise:

Abdominal exercise:

Lower Body exercise:

Full Body exercise:

Set 5

Upper Body exercise:

Abdominal exercise:

Lower Body exercise:

Full Body exercise:

Set 6

Upper Body exercise:

Abdominal exercise:

Lower Body exercise:

Full Body exercise:

1 2 3 4 5 6 7 8 9 10 11 12 13 1

THINK THIN JOURNALS AND DIARIES

Here you will find your own special spaces for you to log all the details you need to keep on track with The New Me Program.

Simply photocopy the number of diary and journal pages you need for the week and keep each day together in a folder. You may even like to cover your folder with some inspirational pictures, quotes or stories of success – forming your own motivational collage.

Food and Exercise Diary

Keeping a food and exercise diary allows you to log your food intake and exercise/activity output so you can make sure you're on track with your calories. Doing this also makes you accountable and gives you insight into your food and fitness choices.

Food diary

By writing down everything that goes into your mouth at the time it goes in and, of course, the amount you have, you're able to monitor your sore spots, identify patterns of struggle, and note things that do and don't work for you – this helps you fast-track what is and isn't working in your diet.

- Write everything you eat at the time of eating – no 'I'll write it down later' or 'I won't write this down because no one will ever know'. This is about you, and for you, so keep it real. You're only lying to, and cheating, yourself if you don't.

- Put everything down, including the time you ate, and what and how much you ate – don't forget little details like a teaspoon of sugar or a spray of cooking oil as it all adds up! Use your calorie-counting book to note down the calories contained.

- Be sure to tally up your total calorie count, per meal, and per day, as you go, so that you can stick to your daily limit and work out your CD (Calorie Deficit).

- You can also use this as a space to note any relevant habits and emotions surrounding your eating habits.

Exercise diary

Writing each bit of exercise you do down can be quite rewarding as you see your good efforts reflected back at you. Keeping these records allows you to keep a true indication of what exercise you're doing, how many calories you're burning as opposed to eating, as well as identifying exercise excuses and finding an exercise plan that works for you and your lifestyle.

- Log the amount of calories burned through planned exercise such as a 30-minute walk, as well as calories burned through incidental activity such as 30 minutes of gardening – remember both types of moving add to your total tally for calories burned each day.

- Be sure to tally up the total calories you burn each day, so you can add this to your BMR (use your BMR x 1.2 for a more accurate figure – refer back to the workshop on page 161), and work out your CD.

- You can also use this space to log workout results such as your heart rate average while working out, how many sets of steps you were able to climb or the distance you made in a 30-minute walk; or any relevant habits and emotions surrounding your activity and exercise habits.

On pages 244 and 245 there is a template that you can use or you can create your own that suits the way you record your information.

My Food and Exercise Diary

Day:

Date:

Food for thought (interesting and inspiring food- and exercise-related thought for the day):

Food				Exercise	
CALORIES IN: Food + Fluids				CALORIES OUT: BMR + Activity + Exercise	
Meals	What? (Description)	How much? (Quantity/ Serving size)	Calories in	What? (Description)	Calories out
Breakfast Time: 7.30am	Egg White Omelette	1 serving	190	30-min walking (moderate pace)	176
Snack Time:					
Lunch Time:					
Snack Time:					
Dinner Time:					
Other Time:					
		Daily total:		Daily total:	

Daily Calories Out | BMR (   ) + Total Calories Out (   ) =

– Daily Calories In | – Total Calories In (   )

Daily Calorie Deficit =

Tip: Make enlarged copies of this template on your photocopier for more room to write your entries.

Water: 🥛 🥛 🥛 🥛 🥛 🥛 🥛 🥛

Today's mood: ☹ 1 2 3 4 5 ☺

Today's hunger levels: 1 2 3 4 5 (5 = most hungry)

Food and Exercise Notes (Thoughts, Excuses Used, Recurring Patterns, Achievements etc): _____

Food and Exercise Goals for tomorrow: _____

Today I am amazing because: _____

My Weekly Weight Loss Forecast

	Daily Calorie Deficits
Monday	
Tuesday	
Wednesday	
Thursday	
Friday	
Saturday	
Sunday	

Weekly Total Calorie Deficit =

Divide by 7700 =

Estimated Weekly Weight Loss =

Note: This is just an estimation; results may vary.

Think Thin Journals

Keeping a journal that logs your thoughts and feelings, as well as creating a space to visualise and manifest your transformation, is an essential part of your weight loss journey.

Feel free to use coloured pencils and textas, and paste inspiring photos or clippings throughout. I encourage you to write in your journal every day, during a quiet time such as first thing in the morning before the kids get up or last thing at night in bed or sitting down next to a lit candle.

Transformation Journal

- This journal is to log your transformation from the old you to The New You, including a space for before and after photographs and your weekly weigh-in results, including your waist measurement and notes on how you feel in a chosen outfit as you lose weight.

*To know and not do
is to truly not know at all.*

Transformation Journal

My Starting Weight: _____

Photos:

PASTE HERE

My Mini Goals:

My Major Goals:

Weekly Weigh-in Log

Day:

Date:

Time:

Weight:

Body fat (if you have body-fat scales or someone to measure this):

Try-on:

Waist measurement:

Other measurements (other sites on your body; resting heart rate; blood pressure; cholesterol; blood sugar; or anything else you want to transform):

The New Me now (note the changes you're noticing in becoming a new person with a new body):

Positive Journal

- The idea of this journal is for when you're down on yourself or wondering why you are bothering with it all, you can look back over your positive journal and realise that you are worth the effort and that you are an absolutely amazing person.

- This journal will help you see what you need to see within yourself when sometimes your vision is blurred.

- Simply write down positive things that you did that day – perhaps you helped somebody, did a workout, took a walk instead of eating, read to your child – as well as positive thoughts, affirmations and things you like about yourself. Now this last part can be hard because we're used to thinking so negatively, but with practice you can gradually change the way you think.

- This is a sacred space for nothing other than positive energy and reinforcement of your positive beliefs about yourself.

- To help build your positive frame of reference, there's a space for you to insert your own daily affirmation. Each day, add a new affirmation: Choose from the list below or write your own.

I am an amazing person.

I have a fantastic goal and I am determined to achieve it.

I can control my choices, so long as I use the determination that I know is inside of me.

To reach my goal weight will mean that I will be able to lead a brilliant life – one of health, joy and happiness.

These foods will still be available when I reach my goal and I am in a state of mind to be able to enjoy them without consequences.

To be in control of what I eat, when I eat and how I feel about my body is a very special feeling.

I prefer the feeling of results rather than the taste of the foods I feel I'm missing.

I am strong, I am determined, I am focused.

I can do this.

I am doing this.

This is easy for me right now.

I love myself and have faith in my achievable goal of losing weight.

This is easy and I will see it through to the end.

Nothing tastes as good as slim feels.

I am in control and I choose to stay focused on the path to success.

I have enough focus and faith in my goal that I will stick to the process of achieving them.

I am beautiful.

I am worth the effort.

I will respond instead of react.

I am an amazing person.

I will look for the positive in everything I do.

I will STAND and BE PROUD.

I am in total control of my life, my emotions and the way that I live my life.

I am happy with who I am.

I will do something today that makes me feel special about being me.

WOW! Imagine how your day would go if it started with you reading these affirmations out loud?

The New Me Positive Journal

Day:

Date:

Daily Affirmation:

_____

_____

Positive thoughts (positive things you did today, positive things you like about yourself, positive steps you made today to lose weight and be healthy):

_____

_____

_____

_____

_____

_____

_____

STICK WITH THE PROGRAM – NO MATTER WHAT!

The final, and most important, part of The New Me Program is to stick with it – no matter what – and never EVER give up. If you veer off the diet or exercise track, this does not give you permission to say, 'I've blown it, I may as well give up'; it does not give you permission to feel you have failed; it does not give you permission to beat yourself up! It is to be seen, and only seen as a step-back, not a setback.

A setback is merely a step-back.

The worst thing you can do is fix damage with damage, so if you're down or you have eaten something you shouldn't have or skipped a workout, then the worst thing you can do is try to fix it by eating more, working out less and beating yourself up. Think of it like this: if you suffer a setback on your journey it is merely one step back; all you need to do to correct it is to take another step forward.

Fair enough, you're not two steps forward like you would have been had you not suffered the setback, but that's fine. The problems only come when you decide to beat yourself up and that means taking another step back, then you eat badly again because you're feeling down (take another few steps back), then you don't go to the gym because you ate badly (take another step back), then you decide you will start again tomorrow as it's late now (take another few steps back), then you decide tomorrow that it's Thursday and you've stuffed your week up now so you may as well start Monday (take even more steps back), then before you know it you are 40 steps back and not in a good position at all. If you had picked up from the initial one step back you would have been back on track and moving forward again, fixing the one step back with one step forward.

Setbacks are merely bumps in the road – they may slow you down, but they don't have to stop you. No matter what setback you encounter you must simply deal with the damage done, put it behind you and move forward; rather than wallowing in self-pity and causing more damage by doing so.

No matter how bumpy your weight loss path is, you need to get back up, dust yourself off and keep going.

And always put things into perspective: you haven't stuffed up a whole diet just because you ate, say, a chocolate bar; all you have done is put yourself a chocolate bar behind as opposed to ruining everything.

There is nothing either good or bad, but thinking makes it so.
– Shakespeare

People ask me every day how I've managed to maintain my weight loss. I am more than happy to let you in on a big secret: **I have maintained my weight loss simply because I have never stopped doing the things that I did that helped me lose weight!**

Through practising my new lifestyle, I got to the point where eating smart, thinking positive and motivating myself to exercise came naturally.

Once you don't have to think about making the right choices, that's when you know you've got it!

Tips for keeping weight off – for good

Most people who have lost weight would attest to the fact that losing the weight wasn't nearly as hard as keeping it off – whether you're just trying to keep off the first kilogram you have lost or a lot of weight, I will leave you with some little tricks and tactics you can use to keep your weight off for good.

- Have a strategy in place. Knowing that you won't be strong every day is the first step in creating a strategy. Have strategies ready to implement while you're of a sound mind before the emotions take over and you're not thinking clearly or rationally. The solution is to always try and hold the next card, to have it in your back pocket, so when you find yourself in a situation you can respond instead of react.

- Always ask yourself, 'Why would I want to add to the emotions by feeling bad about what I've eaten as well as the issues I'm already dealing with?'

- Take control of cravings. Remind yourself that The New Me doesn't eat this way anymore. Once we tell ourselves enough that we can happily get by without certain foods the cravings will subside. Getting to this point takes practice and patience, but you will get there.

- Birthday parties, Easter, Christmas and functions are a part of life, which will tempt you to slip back into bad habits. Just deal with them as they come up, make sensible choices and make up for any binges with extra exercise.

continued

- Keep things varied and fresh. I think plateaus are more a state of boredom than our bodies resisting weight loss: mind gets bored, body gets bored and so we stop doing things that allow us to lose weight. Take a cooking class to learn how to cook a new style of healthy food; try some new recipes; take a new exercise class you've always wanted to try; set new goals that inspire and interest you; dare to take on new challenges and active experiences, such as preparing to do a trek overseas. Remember, repetition leads to boredom. Boredom leads to lack of momentum. Lack of momentum leads to loss of results.

- Experiment with modifying new recipes and creating cooking experiences that fit your new eating style.

- Try a new tactic when things aren't working – this could be embarking on a completely different diet, a new way of working out or maybe working out at a different time of the day.

- Know your triggers. If you come out of an AA program you need to identify the triggers that used to tempt you to take a drink and remove them. The same is true after losing weight.

- Focus on how far you've come. Even if you've only lost 1 kilogram (2.2 pounds), or you're at the end of your weight loss goal, remember that you never have to lose these kilograms again. That's a pretty good feeling, when you think of it this way; knowing you're always getting somewhere. Remember this: 1. So long as you never regain that kilo (pound), then you will never have to lose it again, and 2. If you never stop then I promise you that you will never have to start again or be at the beginning of your weight loss journey. These are two things I am absolutely certain of.

- Perseverance and persistence are the secrets to weight loss. If you stick at it, try different approaches and keep on trying until you work out a solution you will succeed. If you give up, you won't make it – ever. And remember, the journey won't always be hard and full of hurdles you have to keep jumping over. Every time you overcome a setback, you become stronger, you grow, you evolve – and the day will come when the same issue or challenge you struggled with will become so easy to get over when it pops up again you'll probably laugh and wonder why it was so hard in the first place.

- Keep on moving. Understand that you eat every day therefore you should move every day. The need to move does not end when you reach your weight loss goal; it becomes a part of your life for the rest of your life.

- Live the opposite kind of life that caused you to gain weight in the first place.

- When you start to see results this is not an indication for you to go ahead and slack off. No saying, 'Well I've done so well up to now I'll just take a little rest and get back into it soon', or 'I've reached my goal I will stop this and go back to eating normally again'. This approach doesn't work. You need to carry your new healthy habits, your new way of living, your New Me, throughout the rest of your life!

- The best tip to maintain your weight loss is to keep doing what you did to lose weight.

- Remember, the fewer things from your old life you return to doing, the less chance you have of returning to where you were.

A FINAL NOTE

I have shared with you all the tips, tricks and tools I used to lose weight as well as The New Me Program offered at my weight loss retreat. If you go through and put together all of the workshops you have done throughout this book, you would end up with your own User's Guide Workbook to your New Me, offering you a quick reference point to the best plans and strategies for your weight loss; insight into why you failed previously and why you won't fail this time; how much you love and believe in yourself; and, most importantly, your program, diet and affirmations, which set you up to Eat Smart, Move More and Think Thin. You now have my three key elements to successful weight loss and you have your very own solution to your past problem with your weight. Now get to work and it will be behind you forever.

I wish you luck in creating your New Me. If you need help in your journey, or would like support and guidance in following a very low calorie diet to induce safe rapid weight loss, as we do at The New Me Retreat, please feel free to contact me or you may like to visit my team at The New Me Weight Loss Retreat. Or try our online support group and club membership:

visit *www.thenewme.com.au*

or email thenewmeretreat@bigpond.com

or contact The New Me

PO Box 291, Mount Eliza, Victoria 3930, Australia

1800thenewme

Believe in Yourself,

Adro

www.adrohealth.com

A Note on Sources

I have drawn inspiration, motivation and information from many valuable sources on my journey to The New Me, and all of these have helped to shape my philosophy and The New Me program, specifically: My own experience on *The Biggest Loser*; Rhonda Byrne's *The Secret* (Atria Books, 2006), for its powerful reminder of our ability to manifest what we desire and believe we deserve; Eckhart Tolle's *Practicing The Power of Now* (Hodder, 2002), for teaching me how to live in the 'now' (*www.eckharttolle.com*); Stephen C. Lundin's *The Fish Philosophies* (Mobius, 2002) – such an amazing read that really makes you think a little differently about how and what you can control; Ray Kelly for his training knowledge; The Calorie King website (*www.caloricking.com.au*) and pocket book for hours of referencing for the calorie breakdown of the Eat Smart recipes; Celebrity Slim website (*www.celebrityslim.com.au*), which inspired my Exercise and Activity Chart; and Dr John De Martini (*www.drdemartini.com*) for his books and teachings.

The recipes in Part 4 are based on my family favourites and classics with revisions and substitutions that have worked for me and clients at the New Me Retreat; thank you to Samantha Sarnelli for her contribution in developing these recipes with me.

Thank you also to the following for providing me with photographs used in this book: Mac Sarnelli, Matt Quinten, Caroline Garrick, Stuart Bryce, AAP and any old school or family portrait photographers I haven't mentioned from my private collection of shots! Thank you also to all The New Me guests who appear in the photographs featuring the retreat.

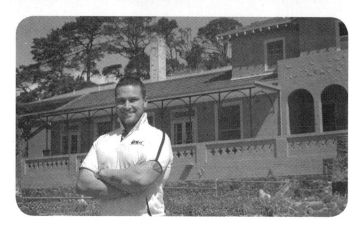

The New Me Weight Loss Retreat is a program created by and inspired by Adro's own weight loss journey, from child- to adulthood. The retreat runs on a 2-week cycle with a minimum 2-week stay and maximum 12-week stay.

The program is based on Adro's philosophy of Eat Smart, Move More, Think Thin – what he believes to be the three key fundamentals for successful weight loss – and is implemented through a variety of practical avenues:

- Tools (starter pack)
- Cooking classes
- Self-cooking
- Group therapy classes
- One-on-one counselling
- Motivation seminars
- Education classes
- Group personal training
- Self-training time
- Dinner outings

Experience the advantages of attending The New Me Weight Loss Retreat:

- Remove yourself from your current sabotaging environment and place yourself somewhere you can't help but lose weight.
- Enjoy the luxury of being able to put yourself first and learn the value of doing so.
- Take the plunge and believe in yourself and discover the power positive affirmation can have on your life.

Find out how amazing it is to have the support of Adro and a retreat filled with people and trainers who have been in exactly the same position as you; to not only find your true self but to learn how to love The New You!

**For bookings and enquiries, please phone 1800 THENEWME,
www.thenewme.com.au or email thenewmeretreat@bigpond.com**